The Problem of Nutrition

Experimental Science, Public Health and Economy in Europe 1914-1945

P.I.E. Peter Lang

Bruxelles · Bern · Berlin · Frankfurt am Main · New York · Oxford · Wien

Josep L. BARONA

The Problem of Nutrition

Experimental Science, Public Health and Economy in Europe 1914-1945

This book has been supported by the Spanish Ministry of Science and Technology [Research Project MICIN HAR2008-0012-E].

1 avenue Maurice, B-1050 Brussels, Belgium
info@peterlang.com; www.peterlang.com

ISBN 978-90-5201-582-8
D/2010/5678/11

Library of Congress Cataloging-in-Publication Data

Barona Vilar, Josep Lluis. The problem of nutrition: experimental science, public health, and economy in Europe, 1914-1945 / Josep L. Barona.
p. cm. Includes bibliographical references. ISBN 978-90-5201-582-8
1. Nutrition--Europe--History--20th century. I. Title.
[DNLM: 1. Nutritional Sciences--history--Europe. 2. History, 20th Century--Europe. 3. International Cooperation--history--Europe. 4. Nutrition Disorders--history--Europe. 5. Public Health--history--Europe. 6. Research--history--Europe. 7. Socioeconomic Factors--Europe. QT 11 GA1 B265p 2010]
TX357.B385 2010 363.8094--dc22 2009050946

CIP also available from the British Library, GB.

Bibliographic information published by "Die Deutsche Nationalbibliothek"
"Die Deutsche Nationalbibliothek" lists this publication in the "Deutsche Nationalbibliografie"; detailed bibliographic data is available on Internet at <http://dnb.d-nb.de>.

Acknowledgements

This book is a result of a research project on nutrition and health during the first half of the 20th century. I have had the opportunity to discuss particular aspects such as the role of international agencies or the rural perspective thanks to conference sessions at Amsterdam, Bergen and Granada. The author is grateful to Mrs. B. Pejovic, archivist of the League of Nations Archives (Geneva), Mr. Fabio Ciccarello and Mr. Giuliano Fregoli, archivists at the Records and Archives Department, FAO (Rome), Dr. Rengenier Rittersma, editor of the journal *Food and History*, Professors Astri Andresen, Tore Grønlie, Josep Bernabeu, Mark Harrison, Ximo Guillem and Enrique Perdiguero for valuable comments and encouragement. Some particular aspects benefited from discussions at the Wellcome Unit for the History of Medicine Oxford and at the Department of Anthropology, History, Cultural Sciences and Religion, University of Bergen, Norway. I want to thank Elisa Cuenca for her support on linguistic revisions.

Contents

CHAPTER 1

Making the Problem of Nutrition in Interwar Years

This book is the result of a research project undertaken in 2005 by a group of Spanish researchers from the Universities of Valencia, Alicante, Miguel Hernández and the Institute of History (High Council for Scientific Research, Madrid). It is focused on the history of nutrition in the 20th century taking Spanish society as the main reference.[1] The project addressed this subject from the perspective of the links between nutrition and health within the context of the outset of the so-called *community nutrition*. My previous research work had concentrated on Spain's participation in the international sanitary movement. In approaching the origin of community nutrition, interactions between the local and the international context emerged as an inescapable referent.[2] In the very complex historical scenery of the first half of the 20th century, interactions between theory and practice, and the local, the national and the international rendered an integrating approach of all such dimensions preferable. Consequently, I decided to orient my investigation toward the analysis of nutrition from a European viewpoint.

The social and economic background

The British historian Eric Hobsbawn has described the first half of the 20th century as the *Age of extremes*, a period of revolutions, crises and conflicts in all realms of social life and in the values and referents that define the human condition.[3] Suffice it to mention the impact of the Great War, the rise of the worker movement and the revolutionary threat – leading to the Bolshevik triumph and the Soviet revolution –, the threat of nationalism and the National Socialist expansion, the clash and tension between the Triple Alliance and the Entente, which divided Europe into two conflicting blocks – the prelude of the Spanish Civil

---

[1] The research project *Nutrición y salud en la España de la primera mitad del siglo XX* was funded by the Spanish Ministry of Health and Education, 2005-2008.

[2] Barona, J.L., Bernabeu-Mestre, J., *La salud y el estado. El movimiento sanitario internacional y la administración española*, Valencia, PUV, 2008.

[3] Hobsbawn, E., *The Age of Extremes, 1914-1991*, London, Abacus, 1995.

War, which in turn constitutes the preamble to the Second World War and the failure of negotiation and pacification policies. All these events drew a landscape of tension, radicalism and political instability – the reflection of waning liberal democracies and rising totalitarian regimes.

In the economic scene, the first decades of the 20th century were also marked by a crisis. To the exceptional circumstances of social conflict typical of pre-war, war and post-war periods, we must add the fiasco caused by the 1929 crash and the great depression of the 1930s, characterised by a deep production crisis in both industry and agriculture, and by the resounding collapse of international trade which all of a sudden transformed the map of wealth, giving way to huge poverty pockets and population changes marked by uncontrolled migrations. This was indeed a dark panorama at a key moment in time for the transformation of the productive system and for women's emancipation and integration into the labour market and, subsequently, for the transformation of family dynamics and roles. As portrayed by Charles Chaplin in *Modern Times*, this period is defined by a shift in the production model boosted by *Fordism* and *Taylorism*, mass production and the access of the average citizen to consumerism and to economic and social life.

Whichever the viewpoint, the first half of the 20th century is a critical, contradictory and essential period to the development of the *civilising process* defined by Norbert Elias as one in which external social constraints proscribing behaviours gradually became internalised; accompanied by feelings of shame directed inward and of repugnance directed towards the others.[4] He suggested that, in modern Western culture, behaviour associated with the body, as it is the case of dietary habits, came to be strictly regulated. The *civilising process* can also be interpreted as the genesis of what Alfons Labisch described as the construction of the *homo hygienicus*,[5] basically an expression of the triumph of the ideals and values of urban bourgeoisies. This was therefore the breeding ground for a new concept of citizenship and the expan-

---

4 Elias, N., *Über den Prozeß der Zivilisation. Soziogenetische und psychogenetische Untersuchungen. Erster Band. Wandlungen des Verhaltens in den weltlichen Oberschichten des Abendlandes* and *Zweiter Band. Wandlungen der Gesellschaft. Entwurf einer Theorie der Zivilisation*, Basel, Verlag Haus zum Falken, 1939 (Published in English as *The Civilizing Process, Vol. I. The History of Manners*, Oxford, Blackwell, 1969, and *The Civilizing Process, Vol. II. State Formation and Civilization*, Oxford, Blackwell, 1982); Andresen, A. *et al.* (eds.), *Citizens, Courtrooms, Crossings*, Bergen, Stein Rokkan Centre for Social Studies, 2008; Barnes, D.S., *The Great Stink of Paris and the Nineteenth-Century Struggle against Filth and Germs*, Baltimore, The Johns Hopkins University Press, 2006.

5 Labisch, A., *Homo Hygienicus. Gesundheit und Medezin in der Neuzeit*, Frankfurt, Campus, 1992.

sion of civil rights, among which hunger, extreme poverty, avoidable disease, infant and birth-related mortality, and the abandonment of children drew a universe of intolerable situations.

That same period also set a milestone in the cultural scene as a key factor for innovation, *modernity* and *progress*. The new bourgeois society boosted urban culture and cosmopolitanism versus the values of countryside living; world exhibitions were fostered in major European cities, art avant-gardes and any art movement breaking away from former conceptions and rules were worshipped, and a new model of universal citizenship was implemented in contrast with the impoverished image of the rural world, one that was growingly considered *backward, non hygienic and rude*, that is to say, little civilised according to urban bourgeoisie standards, and unrefined.[6]

State and international frameworks

It was amidst this complex historical climate that the Interventionist State strongly emerged as a fundamental element in conflict management and stabilisation policies. Bourgeois liberalism and democratic ideals had shifted from 19th century laissez faire attitudes that detested the State to active commitment usually in the form of a *protecting* or *providential State.* The State broke through as a regulating player, a bastion of equity, which regulated social life to prevent abuse, which legitimated itself as the warrantor of common good beyond particular interests – those of the classes or social groups –, which encouraged scientific activity and social care programmes, the construction of hygienic homes and clean schools, and the design of new suburbs. The State emerged as the regulator of inequalities and the main advocate of people's rights. As a result, western countries developed a strong public administration dealing with health, both locally and nationally.

On the other hand, the enormous dimension of social, political and economic problems demanded the configuration of an international framework, one usually employed as a reference for State initiatives. The Treaty of Versailles (1919) outlined a framework for international affairs and the League of Nations did not only foster stabilisation policies focused on trade and political conflicts but also played a determining role in international public health and the appearance of *social medicine*,[7] opening a new period following international sanitary confer-

6 Andresen, A., Barona, J.L., Cherry, S. (eds.), *Making a new countryside? Health Policies and Practices in European History c. 1860-1950*, Frankfurt am Main, Peter Lang, 2009.

7 Weindling, P. (ed.), *International Health Organisations and Movements, 1918-1939*, Cambridge, Cambridge University Press, 1995.

ences and international conferences on hygiene and demography, tuberculosis or infant health. Via international organisations like the Rockefeller Foundation or the Red Cross, international philanthropy reached great relevance in international health on the basis of cooperation between countries.

In this context, nutrition appeared as an excellent ground with multiple dimensions to explore the genesis of experimental knowledge, the social interests involved, and the transfer of knowledge and practices to public health, the economy, trade and politics. The exceptional confluence of all factors influencing the interwar period contributed to building the *problem of nutrition*, the main object of analysis of this book.

Hunger, food and diet

Among the elements with more weight in that construction is the new cultural, social, political and economic significance of hunger, food and diet. Second on the list is the sanitary ideology in force at the time, which closely associated the right to health – an attribute of the new citizenship concept – to the right to decent and sufficient food, arguing that the so-called *organic resistance*, indispensable against infection, was the result of a balanced diet. Consequently, the most unfavoured social groups or those who lived in appalling poverty saw their ability to fight dominant social diseases – like tuberculosis – impaired. A bad diet was considered to be the threshold of infection, and so microbes and foodstuffs drew the attention of physicians and hygienists. We can then understand the interest in identifying deficiency diseases and in defining the concept of deficiency disease, *under-nourishment and malnutrition* according to scientific parameters.

Based on multiple dimensions, the *problem of nutrition* was built during the interwar period. A first aspect to consider is the political and military one, as in time of war preparations as well as during and after the war, it was urgent to ensure a minimum diet for the whole population and, in particular, to avoid famine in certain risk groups: children, mothers, elderly people, the unemployed and the army. Secondly, the economic dimension of the food supply became especially relevant as a result of the deterioration of the global food system, which had been built in the second half of the 19th century. War conflicts and the 1929 crash caused food production and trade to collapse worldwide, with terrible consequences in the 1930s leading to the Second World War. In a purely commercial sense, the crisis of the global food system did not only result in scarcity and a high cost of living but also gave way to protectionism and the return of protection in domestic markets. All such factors encouraged the growing industrialisation of more and more foodstuffs (milk, chocolate, oil, sugar, etc.) as opposed to traditional manufacturing, which made necessary the regulation of production, strict surveillance of fraud and adulteration, and the control of additives, colourings and preservatives. Basically, new rules were needed to stake the boundaries of what was permissible and unacceptable in human diet, a debate whose backdrop was the natural/artificial divide.

The economic, sanitary and political importance of nutrition soon evidenced its cultural dimension. Hygienists and politicians became aware of the deep differences in dietary and cooking habits and traditions between social groups, e.g. between cities and the countryside in the same country, and between European regions. It was necessary to analyse nutritional needs in age groups and for each gender, for manual and factory workers, farmers, and more sedentary professionals. This need prompted field work, surveys, and reports intended to map nutrition and hunger to be used as a basis for political action and social protection.

The new science of nutrition

Scientific knowledge – the new experimental science of nutrition – was to become the cornerstone of a healthy diet and food production. That required solid physiological grounds at the laboratory in relation with calorie coefficients, the need for nutritional principles, foodstuffs values in vitamins and minerals. The parameters of the *optimum diet* and the requirements of the *minimum diet* had to be accurately defined to be able to apply this knowledge to rationing strategies in times of war and scarcity. In turn, the establishment of physiological standards of nourishment had to determine the boundaries of normality and pathology, defining the concepts of food deficiency, under-nourishment and malnutrition.

The figure of the *nutrition expert* stood out in their challenge of establishing physiological, clinical or anthropometric exploration methods to conceptualise and delimit all types of deficiency diseases and malnutrition in children and adults. As nutrition, food availability and hunger stopped being a mere element of natural regulation of the population, they became a cornerstone in economics and politics and an essential part of the process of civilising and disciplining behaviours. In this way, during the interwar period, nutrition opened up an avenue for the medicalisation of diets, the social expansion of medical knowledge and the development of a powerful food industry and international food trade.

In sum, the *problem of nutrition* and the solutions proposed to it were built as a consequence of an imbalance between food production, trade, and demand, since diet habits displayed traditions that were contrary to the new logic of nutrition science and the evolution of the food market.

Once the parameters of the problem of nutrition had been set, a strategy had to be put forward in order to resolve it. Obviously, the answer was to build a new system of scientific knowledge production and to transform social practices; a new culture was needed in food and consumption, in the regulation of what could be eaten, and in the redefinition of the meaning of food. This strategy was mainly promoted by international organisations and by the states both from local and national levels and with a multidimensional focus on the transformation of the food production system, the regulation of industrial production, and the control of quality, fraud, and adulteration.

An important part in this task was played by the League of Nations Health Committee, the International Institute of Agriculture (later FAO), the International Labour Organisation and the Rockefeller Foundation. International trade had to be substantially transformed and the exceptional situation caused by the war confronted. Diet habits also had to be changed on the basis of scientifically defined patterns, and health levels had to be improved by means of a good diet.

The foundations of this new social architecture were found in the onset of a new experimental science of nutrition based on exact physiological concepts that enabled to draw the border between health and pathology. That was the main argument that legitimated experts and the creation of international commissions of nutrition experts and conferences devoted to discuss different aspects of the subject. The brutal aftermath of the world wars and the Spanish Civil War urged an international response and provided an excellent testing ground for the new science of nutrition.

The genesis of the new nutrition knowledge developed between 1920 and 1945, basically taking the following directions:

1. Surveys and reports on diet and food consumption habits in different European countries and on the specific consumption of meat, rice, milk or sugar. They also included studies on specific social groups like pregnant women, children, industrial workers, peasants or the unemployed. This work was supported by international organisations and philanthropic groups.

2. Implementation of public health strategies from national schools of hygiene aimed at training nutrition specialists mainly from health professionals and programming information campaigns for the population to change diet habits. Basically, the goal was to educate according to the principles of nutrition science.

3. Development of an empirical methodology based on the research undertaken by specialists in nutrition analyses, with a dual orientation: social surveys or studies on diet habits and exploration methods. The starting point of the latter was experimental physiology, complemented by anthropometric, clinical and physio-pathological studies. They intended to identify, with scientific-experimental parameters, the nutritional state, deficiency diseases such as beriberi, pellagra, neuropathies due to nutritional deficiencies, and different malnutrition levels.

All that made necessary the validation of an empirical methodology and an agreement concerning the standards of vitamins, minerals, and immediate principles in food and diet. Experimental research was called to lay down the *standards for adequate nutrition*, and a new language emerged from the new science: optimum and minimum diets, protecting and supplementary foods, calorie method, energy coefficient, dietary standards for specific populations, nutritional values, nutritional principles, basal metabolism, calorie requirements, family coefficient scales in rationing.

A large corpus of knowledge started to be developed, used as a starting point for political action and industrial production. As a regulating, stabilising, disciplining and civilising agent, the State – assisted by large international corporations, international agencies and philanthropic organisations – promoted community nutrition policies, trained nutritionist experts, and organised campaigns from the sections of food hygiene and community nutrition of the National Schools of Hygiene and the National Institutes for Mother and Children Care with a view to influencing mothers, who were the main channel of diet information and practices within the family. As of the second half of the 1930s, Institutes of Food Hygiene sprang up across Europe with a view to implementing rationing policies in times of crisis, war and post-war years.

During the interwar period nutrition concentrated a series of aspects that made it an expression of the emergence of experimental knowledge and its transfer into social practices. The nutritional status of the population was not traditionally a matter linked to political economy or state policy. On the contrary, hunger was connected to poverty, and nutritional habits to culture, lacking any moral, social or sanitary implications.[8] It was the advent of the state as a social regulator that placed hunger and feeding at a complex crossroads at which citizenship, cul-

8 Vernon, J., "The Ethics of Hunger and the Assembly of Society: The Techno-Politics of the School Meal in Modern Britain," *American Historical Review*, 110, 2005, p. 693-725.

ture, economy and health played a meaningful role.[9] Food availability became a challenge in many regions for most citizens. Shortages and famines, fears of deprivation and food regulations were a common European experience during the first half of the 20th century. Market and food production, nutrition and conflict stressed the emergence of a global food system starting in the late 19th century, which suddenly experienced a deep crisis during the following years in an era of wars, increasing intervention of the state and raising economic nationalism.

Historiography trends

Historians have traditionally approached food and nutrition in a time of conflict in two main directions. One regards public health and the nutritional state of the population, demographic and epidemiological consequences, expertise and nutritional knowledge from a history of public health perspective.[10] The other historiography trend has focused on agricultural policies, food production and consumption and their influence on the economy, trade and the market.[11] This orientation

---

9 Barona, J.L., "Rural Life and the Problem of Nutrition. Technical Approaches by the Nutrition Committee of the League of Nations," in Andresen, A., Gronlie, T., Ryymin, T. (eds.), *Science, Culture and Politics. European Perspectives on Medicine, Sickness and Health*, Bergen, Stein Rokkan Centre for Social Studies, 2006, p. 201-214; Smith, D. F., Phillips J. (eds.), *Food, Science, Policy and Regulation in the Twentieth Century. International and Comparative Perspectives*, London, Routledge, 2000; Vernon J., 2005; Barona J.L., "Nutrition and Health. The International Context during the Interwar Crisis," *Social History of Medicine*, 21 (1), 2008, p. 87-105.

10 Barona, J.L., "Nutrition, knowledge, and action. International trends and social policies in Spain, 1931-1944," in Andresen, A., Gronlie, T. (eds.), *Transferring Medico-Political Knowledge in 19th and 20th Century Europe*, Bergen, Stein Rokkan Centre for Social Studies, 2007b, p. 91-108; Borowy, I., Grüner, W.D. (eds.), *Facing Illness in Troubled Times. Health in Europe in the Interwar Years 1918-1939*, Frankfurt am Main, Peter Lang, 2005; Cura, M.I. del, Huertas, R., *Alimentación y enfermedad en tiempos de hambre. España, 1937-1947*, Madrid, CSIC, 2007; Kamminga H., Cunningham A., *The Science and Culture of Nutrition (1840-1940)*, Amsterdam, Rodopi, 1997.

11 Caplan, P. (ed.), *Food, Health and Identity*, London, Routledge, 1997; Daunton M., Hilton M. (eds.), *The Politics of Consumption: Material Culture and Citizenship in Europe and America*, Oxford, 2001; Davis R., Wheatcroft S., *The Years of Hunger*, Basingstoke, Palgrave, 2004; Slater, D., *Consumer Culture and Modernity*, Cambridge, 1997; Smith, D.F., "The rise and fall of the Scientific Food Committee during the Second World War," in Smith, D. F., Phillips J., *Food, Science, Policy and Regulation in the Twentieth Century. International and Comparative Perspectives*, London, Routledge, 2000; Steckel, R. H., Rose J. C. (eds.), *The Backbone of History. Health and Nutrition in the Western Hemisphere*, Cambridge, Cambridge University Press, 2002; Trentman F., Just F. (eds.), *Food and Conflict in Europe in the Age of the Two World Wars*, New York, Palgrave, 2006.

includes research into socio-economic factors,[12] standards of living and the role played by food and nutrition and diet,[13] studies of anthropometric indicators such as a synthetic index of well-being or quality of nutritional state,[14] or analyses of the influence of socio-cultural factors, such as body image or the impact of advertising, among others.[15]

These research orientations have led to a greater understanding of the effects of industrialisation, increasing urban growth, or women's entry into the labour force, on changes to the dietary habits of the European population, both rural and urban. In the context of a market economy, the availability of dietary resources varied as a consequence of technological innovation and industrialisation in agriculture, improved productivity in certain areas (oil, wine, fruit and vegetables, factory farming, etc.), or the consolidation of the food industry, among other social factors.

At the same time, diversity of experience and the importance of the local context have been shown to be among the most significant features of this process. In addition to anthropometric studies demonstrating the relationship between height, weight and the environmental conditions which determine nutrition,[16] the differences which have long been observed between the urban and rural setting had to be noted, indicating wider access to food in urban centres. Difficulties were also reported in

---

12 Cussó Segura, X., "Estado nutritivo de la población española, 1900-1970: análisis de las necesidades y disponibilidades de nutrientes," *Revista de Agricultura e Historia Rural*, 36, 2005, p. 329-358; Cussó Segura, X., Garrobou, R., "La transición nutricional en la España contemporánea: las variaciones en el consumo de pan, patatas y legumbres," *Investigaciones de Historia Económica*, 2007, Vol. 7, p. 69-100; Langreo, A., Pujol Andreu, J., "Evolución económica agroalimentaria," in *Como vivíamos: alimentos y alimentación en la España del siglo XX*, Madrid, Lunwerg, 2007, p. 41-66; Nicolau Nos, R., Pujol Andreu, J., "Los factores condicionantes de la transición nutricional en la Europa Occidental: Barcelona, 1890-1936," *Scripta Nova: Revista Electrónica de Geografía y Ciencias Sociales*, 12, 2008, p. 256-265.

13 Simón Pérez, H. J., Escudero, A., "El bienestar en España: una perspectiva de largo plazo, 1850-1991," *Revista de Historia Económica*, 2, 2003, p. 525-566.

14 Martínez Carrión, J.M., "Biología, historia y medio ambiente: la estatura como espejo del nivel de vida de la sociedad española," *Ayer*, 46, 2002, p. 93-122; Martínez Carrión, J.M., "El nivel de vida en la España rural. Siglos XVIII-XX. Nuevos enfoques, nuevos resultados," in Martínez Carrión, J.M., Pérez Castejón, J.J. (eds.), *El nivel de vida en la España rural, siglos XVIII-XX*, Alicante, Universidad de Alicante, p. 15-72.

15 Velasco, C., Rodergas, R., "Los productos alimenticios y la publicidad," in *Como vivíamos: alimentos y alimentación en la España del siglo XX*, Madrid, Lunwerg, 2007, p. 119-138.

16 Beneito, A., Puche Gil, J., "Creixement econòmic i desenvolupament fabril en Alcoi, 1840-1915: Misèria fisiològica sota l'esplendor industrial?," in *La societat industrial al País Valencià*, Alcoi, 2008.

the consumption of animal proteins, in particular of milk and dairy products, in some European regions.[17]

Conflicts over nutrition and food in time of crisis were influenced by traditions, cultural values, social norms, state policies and trade market. The First World War is a breaking point within this background. Food and diet became the site of a dynamic rearrangement between the state and new demanding groups in society. Consumers and civil society were to be linked to social and economic conflict, changing international views and politics.[18]

Consequently, in the interwar years a close relationship between national social reforms and the global rearrangement of the global food system took place, and improvements in food production, and availability, nutritional habits and public health were understood as a part of a global program to eradicate hunger and improve health within the context of the building of a sort of global civil society.[19]

Therefore, since the start of the 20th century, nutrition became a major concern for most European governments, for civil society, workers unions and for other social and charitable organisations. Several factors were central to this process: economic aspects such as food production, food industrialisation and quality control;[20] cultural factors influencing

---

17 Nicolau Nos, R., Pujol Andreu, J., "Variaciones regionales de los precios de consumo y de las dietas en España, en los inicios de la transición demográfica," *Documents de Treball (UAB. Unitat d'Història Econòmica)*, No. 29, 2005.

18 Slater, 1997; Trentman, 2006, p. 6.

19 Trentman, 2006, p. 7.

20 Guillem-Llobat, X., Perdiguero, E., "Fighting adulteration in early European food industrialisation. The case of Alicante (Spain)," in Vámos, É. (ed.), *History of the Food Chain. From Agriculture to Consumption and Waste*, Hungarian Chemical Society, Budapest, 2006a, p. 33-40; Guillem-Llobat, X., "Industrialització i alimentació en la societat valenciana. El control de qualitat dels aliments (1850-1939)," in Herran, N. *et al.* (eds.), *Synergia: Primer Encuentro de Jóvenes Investigadores en Historia de la Ciencia*, Madrid, CSIC, 2006b; Guillem-Llobat, X., "El establecimiento de nuevos límites de calidad para los alimentos en el cambio de siglo (1880-1936)," in Ortiz Gomez, T. *et al.* (eds.), *La Experiencia de enfermar en perspectiva histórica. Actas XIV Congreso de la Sociedad Española de Historia de la Medicina, Granada*, Editorial Universidad de Granada, 2008b, p. 271-274; Guillem-Llobat, X., "El paper dels laboratoris municipals valencians en el control de qualitat dels aliments (1881-1936)," *Actes del Congrès de la Societat Catalana d'Història de la Ciència i de la Tècnica*, 2008c, Vol. 1, p. 293-300; Guillem-Llobat, X., "Food quality controls in the European Periphery. Valencian scientists and laboratories in the late nineteenth century," in Simon, J. *et al.* (eds.), *Beyond Borders: Fresh perspectives in history of science.* Cambridge Scholars Publishing, Cambridge, 2008d, p. 301-324.

local dietaries mainly in rural districts;[21] scientific research propelled by the discovery of the physiological basis of nutrition.[22]

A new international landscape was shaped during the interwar period. Nutrition – as health itself – became an essential factor for social stability as a sort of ground for the making of citizenship, implying changing relationships between state, society and individuals. The provision of food became a basic human right and a problem to challenge, endowed with a moral dimension. Nevertheless, accordingly to the new scientific ideas, traditional production schemes – mainly in agriculture – and dietary habits could have negative effects on both health and the economy. Under the pressure of the war and the economic crisis, food production and consumption increasingly became a state concern and a political issue.

This book offers a general approach to several dimensions of the problem of nutrition during the interwar years, trying to show how diet and food availability became a central issue for the economy, scientific research, politics and health in the international agenda, a subject widely discussed in international organisms and conferences. It adds a general overview to previous research mainly focussed on specific aspects and countries.[23] The scientific, political and economic dimensions of nutrition allowed politicians and experts to dream of a rational solution to the problem through the design of minimum and optimum standard diets for different income groups, professions and ages. The problem I want to wrestle with in this book is how international organisations contributed to boosting experimental science and to shaping public health expertise on nutrition, and how they tried to influence food production and dietary habits. The effects of the war and the devastating landscape of malnutrition in internment camps show the failure of the strong international commitment.

Due to the intervention of the League of Nations, the International Labour Organisation and the International Institute of Agriculture (Food and Agriculture Organisation as from 1948), expert commissions shaped an international context influencing governments, scientists, economists and food producers to cope with the problem of nutrition. International agencies promoted technical surveys on the nutritional state of the population in countries and regions, commissioned experts' conferences

---

21 Barona, 2006a; Kamminga, Cunningham, 1997.

22 Barona, 2008a, 2008b.

23 Kamminga, Cunningham, 1997; Steckel, R.H., Rose, J.C., *The Backbone of History. Health and Nutrition in the Western Hemisphere*, New York, Cambridge University Press, 2002; Vernon, 2005.

to implement international standards aiming to improve the physiological knowledge of nutrition, and screened rural diet and nutritional habits in Europe.[24] International political economists and economy historians have mainly examined the problem in terms of the power of interest groups or state strategy,[25] but the role of the international organisations in the impulse of experimental science and health policies – the major dimension of the problem – have been scarcely considered.[26]

War and post-war years were a decisive period in the appearance of a new international vision of coordination in many aspects of state intervention. Rather than protectionist-state centred politics and liberal market-based traditions, an alternative emerged connecting elements of the civil society with mechanisms of global governance including a vision of mutual dependence. Historiography has shown that since the end of the 19th century, European countries showed different traditions regarding the global food system. Britain had a predominant free trade tradition, quite different from protectionist Germany, France and Russia, far from more simple and self-sufficient agricultural communities in the Mediterranean countries, while other countries were more market and export oriented, like Sweden, Denmark, Belgium, Netherlands and Switzerland.[27]

Therefore, the role of expert scientists would not only influence knowledge, but also inspire agricultural and health policies, and participate in education and propaganda programmes to civilise and change habits. Around nutrition and health a wide program of intervention was shaped aiming at disciplining, civilising and changing production and consumption patterns and popular habits. The emergence of nutrition and hunger as a problem contributed to the recognition of the social dimension of the self through the emergence of international and state social policies. Hunger, feeding and famine appeared as a threat and therefore they became a central locus of action for social and political stability, change programmes and modernisation. Around the social and scientific transformation of nutrition, local and international experts appeared, becoming principal agents for the development of public health and social welfare policies.

The emergence of nutrition as a scientific, medical and political locus was closely connected to market and consumption, but also to cultural and socio-historical factors and to the emergence of the state as

24 Barona, 2008a.

25 Trentmann, 2006, p. 14.

26 Weindling, 1995.

27 Trentmann, 2006, p. 15.

a social regulator. The international crisis and the changing meaning of hunger and poverty as unacceptable social realities on the one hand, and the emergence of new governmental responsibilities on the other were some of the most meaningful factors.[28] As early as in the second half of the 19th century, social initiatives, such as school meals, charity meals for the poor, mothers and industrial workers, propaganda campaigns on dietary habits, experimental research on physiology of nutrition, and economic and agricultural policies were all put in place in order to fight hunger as an intolerable reality. No specific political ideology monopolised this social and scientific process which indeed was more broadly related to the general value of progress and modernity widely spread in most Western societies.[29]

The new social ethics confronted hunger with practical actions in order to determine optimum standard diets, reshape dietary habits, plan agricultural production, implement rationing policies, design school and family meals, and discipline citizenship habits via campaigns. Hunger and feeding were no longer considered purely private matters because diet became a locus for experimental research, a scientific field of knowledge and a practice associated with health and disease, all these aspects being responsibilities for the state. Both for national and international organisations, the *problem of nutrition* encompassed public and individual health, working conditions, agriculture production, clinical screening, social stability and scientific research.[30]

During the late 1920s and the 1930s, the new culture of nutrition and its health dimension (optimum diet, dietary standards, undernourishment, malnutrition) fully emerged into the international sphere.[31] Scientific patterns of feeding and cultural habits were faced. Physiology of nutrition was considered to contribute more than merely nutritional benefits, for, according to the new mentality, experts and authorities believed that the diet was to be adapted to scientific patterns as a way of improving human development from a eugenic perspective and overcoming long-standing shortcomings and superstitions.[32] In the opinion of

---

28 Andresen, Grønlie, Ryymin (eds.), 2006 and 2007; Baldwin, P., *The Politics of Social Solidarity. Class Bases of the European Welfare State 1875-1975*, Cambridge, Cambridge University Press, 1990.

29 Vernon, 2005; Hendrick, H., *Child Welfare. Historical Dimension, Contemporary Debate*, Cambridge, Polity Press, 2003.

30 *Problem of nutrition. Interim Report of the Mixed Committee on the Problem of Nutrition*, 3 vols., Geneva, League of Nations, 1936. [A.12.1936.II.B].

31 Burnet, E., Aykroyd, W.R., 'Nutrition and Public Health," *League of Nations Quarterly Bulletin of the Health Organisation*, 1935, Vol. 4, No. 2, p. 323-474.

32 Carrasco Cadenas, E., *Ni gordos, ni flacos. Lo que se debe comer*, Madrid, Diana, 1935; Burnet, Aykroyd, 1935.

scientists, public health experts and politicians, the science of nutrition was to have a civilising effect upon the population, mainly workers and peasants, mothers and children. Knowledge on nutrition was to become legitimated by science and expertise, to be spread from the laboratory to the school, hospital, factory and the home, to influence food production, improve and rationalise the economy, shape scientific knowledge and become a technical tool for future generations. As a material instrument of statecraft, nutrition was a tool of power and some European politicians were determined to use it. Indeed, nutritional knowledge had to become quantifiable so that political and scientific initiatives could challenge the international crisis.

Nutrition and public health

According to J. George Harrar, President of the Rockefeller Foundation in the interwar years, the discovery of the calorie as a unit of measurement had led directly to an "informal alliance" of "scientists, farmers, government agencies, educators, and processors" working to fight malnutrition worldwide.[33] The *problem of nutrition* pooled, in its public health dimension, national and international efforts during the interwar period mainly through the activities of the League of Nations' Health Committee, often working co-ordinately with national schools of health in several European countries in the 1930s with the support of the Rockefeller Foundation and the collaborative expertise of the International Institute of Agriculture.

Hunger and poverty reinforced their social and public health dimensions in most European countries already during the second half of the 19th century.[34] Consequently the state participated in the regulation of social relations affecting labour legislation, the protection of mothers and children, promoting health and sanitary campaigns, and school reforms from a hygienist perspective. School medical inspection and school canteens became a component of the new state policies on social reforms for human improvement through feeding. Summer camps not only aimed the contact with healing nature, but also feeding undernourished low class children. The first municipal institution for school medical inspection was created in Brussels in 1878.[35] In 1883, a medical school service was set up in Paris, which then spread to other French provinces. Finally, a national Act created the French League for School

---

33 Cullather, 2007, p. 5.

34 Baldwin, 1990; Maurer, D., Sobal J. (eds.), *Eating Agendas: Food and Nutrition as Social Problems*. New York, 1995; Sen, A.K., *Poverty and Famines. An Essay on Entitlement and Deprivation*, Oxford, Oxford University Press, 1981; Vernon, 2005.

35 Barona, 2007b.

Hygiene (1903). The First International Conference on School Hygiene was held in Nuremberg (1904), a Second Conference in London (1906) and also in Paris (1906). In April 1912, the First Spanish Conference on School Hygiene took place in Barcelona. It defined the inalienable rights of children, set up a *Liga de Higiene Escolar* [School Hygiene League], and requested the extension of medical inspection at schools. The health-at-school policy also comprised school meals and canteens, which emerged in Europe from the 1860s onwards in the context of broad debate on compulsory education and an environment in which hunger and its links with health was becoming far more visible.[36]

A second dimension of nutrition in the context of public health comes from the idea that good nutrition is essential to enjoying an optimum health status, a condition necessary to fight infectious diseases, indeed the main health problem during the first half of the 20th century. Feeding was to be considered the basis of good body development and a healthy state, a source of organic energy, something fundamental in front of the threat of consumption. The so-called organic energy was considered to be essential to the understanding of the spread of infectious diseases such as tuberculosis. The concept of the pre-tubercular condition in children as a predisposition to the disease related to defective feeding, excessive work, a lack of hygiene and poor living conditions.[37] These elements cause us to argue that before the emergence of nutrition as an experimental scientific research field especially in the 1930s, hunger and feeding became a subject for social action mainly associated with public health and an optimum health status in order to minimise the risk of suffering infectious diseases. This stage was prior to the emergence of a new science of nutrition based on vitamins, organic elements and specific deficiency diseases.[38] The concept of *organic resistance* to infection was directly related to nutritional state and optimum diet. Poor nutrition was claimed to be the main factor for impaired organic resistance as a previous stage leading to infection. This was particularly accepted in the case of tuberculosis. From this perspective, vaccines and medicines were important in fighting tuberculosis and other infectious diseases, and also in preventing contagion. But this was

36 Hendrick, 2003.

37 Ryymin, T., "Tuberculosis-threatened Children. The Rise and Fall of a Medical Concept, *c.* 1900-60," in Andresen A., Grønlie T., Ryymin T. (eds.), *Transferring Medico-Political Knowledge in Nineteenth- and Twentieth-Century Europe*, Bergen, Rokkan Centre for Social Studies, 2007; Ryymin T., "Tuberculosis-threatened Children. The Rise and Fall of a Medical Concept in Norway, *c.* 1900-60," *Medical History*, 2008, Vol. 52, p. 347-364.

38 Barona, 2008a; Barona, 2008b.

no more important than a good nutritional condition, which was considered to be the basis of a good treatment of any infection. In the late 1920s, poverty, the problem of children's health and infectious diseases, and the economic crisis paved the road for a new milestone, namely the big international boost of scientific research on nutrition.

CHAPTER 2

Nutrition and Public Health: the International Response

The Great War represented a milestone in the process of nutrition becoming a matter of concern in the international sphere. Its political, demographic and economic consequences during the following decades were an immense threat to international stability. Food had already been included in the agenda of international meetings of experts and social movements before the First World War, stretching from malnutrition, feeding of children and pregnant women, relief to adulteration and the search for a healthy, balanced diet. In the 1920s there was a shift away from charitable relief to a more professionalised and scientific approach to nutrition and infectious diseases' relief. The International Labour Organisation [ILO] and the League of Nations' Health Organisation placed the emphasis on scientific knowledge and became international transmitters of new nutritional knowledge as well as sites from which reformers put pressure on their national governments to raise minimum standards and social benefits.[1] As Trentmann states:

> Food was no longer just a relative marker of different degrees of civilisation or a symbol of national identity, as in pre-war contrasts between the white and the black loaf, but an essential good with universally applicable standards of optimal health. Or put differently, different societies became part of the same universal frame of analysis, where individuals and groups could be lined up against the same measuring road of optimal nutritional standards.
>
> [...] The universal standards of nutrition and the international model of trade coordination provided a shared mental space for East and West. Where imperial food politics had been characterised by hierarchical distance and political asymmetry (civilised versus less civilised; the sender versus the recipients of charity; responsible empire and debt-ridden victim), global food politics moved towards a greater sense of equivalence: malnutrition was a universal problem; trade regulation required adjustments from both consuming and producing nations; domestic welfare required global awareness and action.[2]

---

1 Trentmann, 2006, p. 29-30.

2 Trentmann, 2006, p. 39.

International agencies and technical reports

Since its foundation, the League of Nations got involved in the prevention and control of disease. Its Council drew up a scheme for a Health Organisation as soon as in February 1920. Several steps forward led to the constitution of a Health Committee (Geneva, August 1921) and a co-operative strategy with the *Office International d'Hygiène Publique*, in Paris, the International Labour Organisation [ILO] and the International Institute of Agriculture [IIA], in Rome.[3] A *Health Committee*, an *Advisory Council*, and a *Health Section of the Secretariat* constituted a complex administrative framework devoted to the coordination of an ambitious program in international health. The series of *Annual Reports*, the *Bulletin of the Health Organisation*, the *Annual and Monthly Epidemiological Reports*, the *Weekly Epidemiological Records* (Geneva), and the *Weekly Fasciculus* (Singapore) summarised the main trends of intense activity in international health.[4]

The first technical reports by the Health Organisation of the League of Nations date back to 1926, with a wide range of documents on nutrition-related aspects.[5] All of them emphasised the importance of developing a science of nutrition as a point of departure to challenge the nutritional requirements of the global population. These scientific studies had to have both a social and experimental orientation, and include standardising methods to study dietary needs, the links between nutrition, agriculture, the economy and public health especially in rural areas, statistics in countries and regions, as well as reports on the real feeding restrictions in Europe and the diseases caused by them. Meaningful players such as John Maynard Keynes, Jean Monnet and

---

3 Dubin, M., "The League of Nations Health Organization," in Weindling, P. (ed.), *International health organisations and movements, 1918-1939*, Cambridge, Cambridge University Press, 1995, p. 56-80.

4 A summary of the activities developed by the League of Nations can be found in "Bibliography of the Technical Work of the Health Organisation of the League of Nations, 1920-1945," *League of Nations Bulletin of the Health Organisation*, 1945, Vol. 11, p. 6.

5 Boxes in the Archive of the League of Nations (Geneva) containing specific information on nutrition include R.6133 to R.6140. Some internal reports related to the period 1928-1937 (R.5865-5866) are devoted to nutrition. See also Saiki T., *Necessity of the Study of Nutrition*, Geneva, League of Nations, 1927. Document R.5910 analyses food supplies, reparation and distribution (1929). It included also some other internal documents on food supplies: preparations alleged to contain vitamins (1929-1932) and food supplies, standardisation of vitamins (1930-1932) (Documents R.5921 y R.6078-79). Documents R.5935 and R.6009 (1932) were entirely devoted to food supplies, production and distribution of vitamin standards. Document R.5936 contains an *Étude de l'état alimentaire* (1932-3) and also several *Études sur la meilleure utilisation, pour l'alimentation des budgets réduits* (1932-1933).

Albert Thomas, all advocated intervention in food production and consumption as one of the best alternatives to face economic instability.

Most of the technical and social studies of nutrition during the 1920s and 1930s focused on European countries (Czechoslovakia, Denmark, France, Great Britain, Hungary, The Netherlands, Romania, Spain, Portugal and Sweden).[6] Europe was the centre of the crisis. War consequences, international conflicts and financial chaos could explain a concern basically focused on European regions. But the nutritional situation of South Africa, Chile, China, India, Japan and the Philippines was also reported in the League of Nations' conferences.

In the fight against deficiency diseases and malnutrition, special attention was paid to the protection of basic foodstuffs, such as milk, bread, meat and rice, subject to technical approaches that analysed the nutritional value of the principles contained and dietary needs at every stage of life. The emergence of a science of nutrition, grounded on experimental principles implied, on the one hand, expertise based on new methods and, on the other, technologies to survey and evaluate the nutritional condition of the population and its impact on public health. Moreover, it required political measures to rearrange agriculture, commercial networks and education and to change the population's habits.

The huge impact of malnutrition and deficiency diseases associated to dietary problems during the post-war years gave scientific authority to nutritionists more and more endowed with a scientific approach based on experimental research about bodily energy needs and on the physiological contribution of vitamins, minerals, proteins, carbohydrates and fats. Politicians and economists turned their eyes to the new science of nutrition as a starting point of a steady solution.

As of the mid 1920s the Health Organisation of the League of Nations got engaged in the study of nutrition in relation to public health as an international problem requiring attention from a variety of

---

6 Milk and Milk Products in Sweden (Studies on nutrition), 1926, (Document C.H./Com.Exp.Alim./5: Divers/I); Moerkeberg, H.C. *Meat inspection in Denmark and Inspection of Milk in Danemark*, 1924, C.H./E.P.S./49; Mackenzie, M.D., "The Administrative Machinery by which the Adequate Nourishment of the Poor is Ensured in Great Britain," *League of Nations Quarterly Bulletin of the Health Organisation*, 1933, Vol. 2, p. 333-352; [McDougall, E.J.] "Rural dietaries in Europe," *Bulletin of the Health Organisation*, 1939, Vol. 8, No. 3, p. 470-497. [C.H./Com.Exp.Alim./59, 25 p.]; Muehel, W., "Ill effects of food restrictions in Europe, 1940-1944," *League of Nations Bulletin of the Health Organisation*, 1945-1946, Vol. 12; *Nutrition in various countries*, Series of League of Nations Publications, Geneva, 1936. [Technical Report A.12(b).1936.II.B]; "Report on Bread in several European Countries," *League of Nations Bulletin of the Health Organisation*, 1939, Vol. 8, p. 498-555.

perspectives. In 1925 a proposal from the Yugoslavia delegation to the Assembly of the League of Nations requested the Health Committee to study "the methods to be recommended in the interests of public health for the regulation of the manufacture and of the sale of food products." Shortly after, in 1926, the Health Organisation published a collection of memoranda on the physiology of nutrition and its clinical meaning.[7] In 1927 the specialist on physiology of nutrition T. Saiki gave several lectures on nutrition in the USA, Argentine, Brazil and Chile under the auspices of the League of Nations. In 1926 and 1927 the League of Nations' Health Organisation promoted a visit by Egerton Grey, a professor at the University El Cairo, to Tokyo, who published an internal report about *The Food of Japan* following the visit.[8]

During the 13th session of the Health Committee held in 1928, Léon Bernard, on behalf of the French Government, asked for nutrition to be included into the Committee's work programme. As we know, the situation became more urgent and dramatic as from the following year. Based on its interest in nutrition, in 1931 a collective tour of the Health Committee to the USA took place in order to study the supply of milk; a year later, in 1932, the Government of Chile requested collaboration from the League of Nations to carry out a study of popular nutrition in Chile.

In 1932, general concerns grew about the consequences of the crisis and, as a result, the 19th session of the Health Committee undertook a study on the effects of the economic crisis on public health, with particular reference to the under-nourishment conditions caused by the recession. Two conferences of experts were convened in connection with the studies on nutrition. The first one was the Experts Conference held in Rome in September 1932 and the second one was held in Berlin in December 1932. We shall refer to them in a further chapter, but let us now advance that in the backdrop of these two conferences a call was implicit to experimental science and technical expertise to consider the principles of an adequate diet as a means to overcome the economic crisis.[9]

The problem of nutrition was in 1932 fully integrated in the international agenda due to exceptional circumstances. In accordance with the recommendation of the Berlin Conference and the invitation of the

7 Saiki T., *Progress of the Science of Nutrition in Japan*, Geneva, League of Nations, 1926. It was followed by Saiki, 1927.

8 *The Food of Japan*. Internal report. Archive of the League of Nations Doc CH 861.

9 Information about these conferences in *Quarterly Bulletin of the League of Nations*, Vol. I., 1932-1933, No. 3 and Vol. II, 1933, No. 1.

Council of the League of Nations, the Health Organisation and the International Labour Organisation combined their efforts to study the most suitable methods for safeguarding the public health during the time of depression. A Joint Conference of Experts in Sanitary Administration and Social Insurance promoted by the League of Nations and the International Labour Organisation, including members from Belgium, the United Kingdom, Czechoslovakia, France, Germany, the United States of America and Yugoslavia, met on two occasions under the chairmanship of M.G. Cahen-Salvador, State Councillor, Paris. Discussions on those international meetings were summarised in a further report.[10]

A couple of years later, in September 1935, the General Assembly of the League of Nations having considered the subject of nutrition in relation to public health and the effects of improved nutrition on the consumption of agricultural products, urged Governments to examine the practical means of securing better nutrition and invited the Health Organisation to continue and extend its work on nutrition in relation to international public health.[11] Furthermore it requested the Council to instruct the technical organisation of the League of Nations, in consultation with the International Labour Office and the International Institute of Agriculture, to collect, summarise and publish information on the measures taken in all countries for securing improved nutrition. The Assembly also proposed to appoint a Committee, including agricultural, economic and health experts, instructed to submit a general report on the whole question, in its health and economic aspects.[12]

Some months before, in June 1935, the 19th session of the ILO had voted unanimously a resolution recognising that adequate nutrition was essential for the workers well-being and their families. At the same time the resolution recognised that in many countries large numbers of persons were not sufficiently nourished. The ILO resolution stated that an increasing of consumption of agricultural foodstuffs would help to raise standards of life and relieve the depression in agriculture. The ILO Conference requested the Governing body to continue investigations in collaboration with Health and Economic Organisations of the League of Nations, the IIA and others.

---

10 "Report of the Health Organisation for the Period October 1932 to September 1933. IV. Economic Depression and Public Health," *League of Nations Quarterly Bulletin of the Health Organisation*, 1933, Vol. 2, p. 529-535.

11 *The Problem of Nutrition. Interim Report of the Mixed Committee on the Problem of Nutrition*, Geneva, Series of League of Nations Publications, 1936. [Technical Report A.12.1936.II.B].

12 *The Problem of Nutrition*, 1936, p. 7-8.

As a consequence of the international organisations' agreement on the wide dimension of the problem and the necessity of collaboration, a mixed technical commission was founded which held in London in November 25th-29th, 1935. The mixed commission had to prepare a "Report on the Physiological Basis of Nutrition."[13] This report had a preliminary character including a general assessment about the problem of nutrition, embodying the suggestions made by the Mixed Committee to the Assembly and giving a general idea of the problems involved. Three more volumes reported on the physiological basis of nutrition according to the Technical Commission of the Health Committee, on the state of nutrition in various countries, summarizing the available data delivered by governments replying the Secretary-General's Circular letter of November 30th, 1935. It contained a survey of popular dietaries since the war and a summary of statistical materials. The last part contained statistics of food production, consumption and prices in several countries.

Provided that the Mixed Committee included experts representing not only the League of Nations, but also the International Labour Office and the International Institute of Agriculture, we might conclude that access to foodstuffs and nutrition was given international priority in policies and relationships in the 1930s. Some of its general recommendations have been mentioned above. The Mixed Committee showed special concern about what steps should be taken to meet nutritional need of the lower-income sections of the community – children and the unemployed – to ensure the adequate food supply, especially protective foods at prices within the reach of all social groups. A main challenge was the necessity to safeguard the interests of producers as cornerstone of the system. Therefore improving marketing and distribution of foodstuffs and reducing their costs both in the cities and in industrial and rural areas was necessary, encouraging collaboration between co-operatives and other forms of producers' and consumers' organisations.

E. Burnett and W.R. Aykroyd's report

In 1934, in view of the social importance of nutrition and as a consequence of the work done, the Health Committee, which was then preparing a three-year programme, entrusted E. Burnet and W.R. Aykroyd a series of enquiries in different countries such as the United Kingdom, France, the United States of America, Denmark, Sweden, Norway and

13 "Report on the Physiological Bases of Nutrition by the Technical Commission of the Health Committee in the meeting held in London 25-29 November 1935," *League of Nations Quarterly Bulletin of the Health Organisation*, 1936, Vol. 5, No. 3, p. 391-415.

the Union of Soviet Socialist Republics, on special aspects related to public health and the role played by institutions linked to nutrition policies in these countries.[14] The report emphasised on each page the importance of international economic conditions and income differences across social groups in relation to adequate nutrition. A simple sentence serves as an example to summarize its philosophy: "The general problem of nutrition as it presents itself today is that of harmonising economic and public health development."[15]

The report by Burnet and Aykroyd was published at a time when the social problems of housing and nutrition were definitely occupying the foremost position in public health. Continuing the work carried out by the Rome and Berlin Conferences, the report thereby addressed the preoccupations arising out of the protracted economic depression. It seems to me that what should be underlined is the fact that the report contained the essential elements for a general discussion of the practical problems of nutrition in relation both to public health and to economic recovery. It was thereby a natural consequence that it should be used as a basis of discussion when the delegations of twelve Governments at the sixteenth Assembly of the League, held in September 1935, requested that nutrition should be placed on the agenda.

Indeed, the discussion in the Second Committee of the Assembly was introduced by Mr. Bruce, the Australian delegate, who stressed in his intervention the necessity for marrying agriculture and public health in the interests of the latter. An increasing consumption of protective foods was presented as a remedy for malnutrition and as some help to face the agricultural crisis. Bruce claimed for a change in State protective subsidies, so that they could serve to increase consumption rather than to restrict production.

Lord de la Warr, a representative of the United Kingdom delegation, presented a report to this meeting of the Assembly considering the subject of nutrition in relation to public health and of the positive effects of improved nutrition on the consumption of agricultural products in such a difficult context. Consequently, the Assembly of the League of Nations adopted the following resolution:

> The Assembly, having considered the subject of nutrition in relation to public health and of the effects of improved nutrition on the consumption of agricultural products, urges Governments to examine the practical means of securing better nutrition and requests the Council:

---

14 E. Burnet and W.R. Aykroyd report was summarised at the *Quarterly Bulletin of the League of Nations*, 1935, Vol. 4, No. 2, p. 323-474.

15 Burnet, Aykroyd, 1935, p. 394.

1. To invite the Health organisation of the League of Nations to continue and extend its work on nutrition in relation to public health;

2. To instruct the technical organisations of the League of Nations, in consultation with the International Labour Office and the International Institute of Agriculture, to collect, summarise and publish information on the measures taken in all countries for securing improved nutrition and

3. To appoint a Committee, including agricultural, economic and health experts, instructed to submit a general report on the whole question, in its health and economic aspects, to the next Assembly, after taking into consideration, *inter alia*, the progress of the work carried out in accordance with paragraphs above.[16]

At the same time, the International Labour Office, which had been informed of the general plan of action contained in the Burnet and Aykroyd report, gave proof of its interest in a collaborative participation. The Mixed Advisory Agricultural Committee, a board which ensured liaison and co-operation between the ILO and the International Agricultural Institute of Rome (IIA), and the International Committee for Inter-co-operative Relations, which was a private organisation for liaison between agricultural and consumers' co-operatives, under the chairmanship of the Director of the ILO, had expressed their desire to co-operate in studying the question of the nutrition of workers. Therefore, at the beginning of 1930 a network of international organisations agreed on the search for expertise to face the crisis, taking the population's nutrition as a main tool.

In 1930, the Polish expert of the League of Nations Health Committee, Witold Chodzko, Head of the National School of Hygiene in Warsaw, summed up existing fears regarding the poor nutritional conditions in the rural areas of most European countries.[17] A month later, the League of Nations Health Committee appointed a Sub-Committee on Rural Health, consisting of the Spanish expert Gustavo Pittaluga, as president, Witold Chodzko, Gerard Fitzgerald, Carl Hamel, Alberto Lutrario, Ludwik Rajchman and Frank Boudreau. They represented most of the national schools of health in European countries, where public health experts established links with national public health policies.

When the 19th International Labour Organisation Conference was held in June 1935, attention was drawn to the problems of nutrition in the report by the Director of the Organisation, and in statements by Sir Frederick Stewart, Miss Paterson and Miss Grace Abbot, government

16 Burnet, Aykroyd, 1935, p. 395.

17 Chodzko, 1930.

delegates of Australia, New Zeeland and the United States of America, respectively. At the end of the conference the following resolution was unanimously adopted:

> Seeing that adequate nutrition, both in quantity and in quality, is essential to the health and well-being of the workers and their families;
>
> And seeing that, in various countries, evidence has been brought forward to show that large numbers of persons both in town and country are not sufficiently or suitably nourished;
>
> Seeing, moreover, that an increase in the consumption of agricultural foodstuffs would help to raise standards of life and relieve the existing depression in agriculture:
>
> The Conference welcomes the attention drawn by the Director in his report to the problem of nutrition and requests the Governing Body to instruct the Office to continue its investigation of the problem, particularly in its social aspects, in collaboration with the Health and Economic Organisations of the League of Nations, the International Institute of Agriculture and other bodies capable of contributing to its solution, with a view to presenting a report on the subject to the 1936 session of the Conference.[18]

Nutrition was present in every international event. During the 22nd session of the Assembly of the League of Nations held in October, 1935, the Health Committee considered Burnet and Aykroyd's report and discussed the hygienic aspects of the problem, recommending the circulation of the report among national administrations. Political and sanitary measures pointed out the necessity for educating medical practitioners, public health workers and the public in the field of nutrition. A resolution was adopted, asking the Technical Commission on Nutrition to select a list of questions, to be classified by order of priority, as a basis for the work to be carried out in co-operation with the other international institutions mentioned above.

The members of the Technical Commission on Nutrition that were appointed were A. Durig (Austria), E.P. Cathcart, E. Mellanby and J.B. Orr (United Kingdom), M.J. Alquier, A. Mayer and L. Lapicque (France), F. Bottazzi (Italy), A. Höjer, C. Schiötz and L.S. Fridericia (Scandinavian States), B. Sbarsky (USSR), E.V. McCollum, M. Swatz Rose and W. Sebrel (USA). H. Chick (London) was invited to participate, since he was the technical secretary of the International Conference on Standardisation of Vitamins.

---

18 Burnet, Aykroyd, 1935, p. 395-396.

Public health, physiology and clinical knowledge

The League of Nations' Health Committee had set up an Advisory Commission on Nutrition in 1932, which was supposed to face the most important challenges: to work under scientific patterns, limits and definitions of malnutrition; to promote the standardisation of methods used in dietary studies, and to establish optimum and minimum diet standards according to the physiological contribution of vitamins, minerals, fats, carbohydrates and protein requirements. Such big commitments were to be accompanied by other challenges such as the discussion of guiding principles for a healthy human diet; the spread of clinical methods to determine the state of nutrition in school children; the establishment of patterns of nutritional requirements at all ages; the identification of specific diets for those sectors of the population on small incomes, and the implementation of surveys on the state of nutrition in every country, particularly in rural areas. This was an ambitious and long-term programme requiring technical and methodological agreement among all the active countries in the League of Nations' Health Committee. The international response promoted by the League of Nations required as, a first condition, the creation of a fully legitimated international group of experts. Then, a series of meetings, conferences, technical documents, scientific articles and regional surveys would produce an assessment of the situation as a point of departure for further strategies based on the coordination of national and international action.[19]

It was hoped that, following the dissemination of the new scientific knowledge about nutrition and its influence on social practices, substantial changes would take place in all the aspects implied. Nutrition would be considered one of the main fields requiring technical expertise and political action to deal with health and solve social problems originated as a consequence of the economic recession, international conflicts and the war and post-war crisis.

The Final Report of the Mixed Committee of the League of Nations on Relation of Nutrition to Health, Agriculture and Economic Policy (1937) marked the culmination of the nutritional programme against international under-consumption. Increasing the consumption of "protective" foods was a dual strategy to tackle malnutrition and agricultural depression. This reference report stressed the need for governments to give a lead in raising public knowledge of nutrition and established the centrality of consumption for global trade and agriculture improvement:

---

19 *Introductory note on the work accomplished (History and method)* by the League of Nations up to October 1935 (Nutrition), 12 p.

> The more recent advances in medical science have established the fact that physical inferiority is largely due to imperfect nutrition [...] At the same time, the discoveries of the last thirty years leading to the newer knowledge of nutrition show with ever increasing certainty that inadequate nutrition plays an excessive proportion of underdeveloped school-children and adolescents and the poor health and small output of a large number of workers. Deficiencies in diet and diseases of nutritional origin can be observed, not only among urban populations, but also among dwellers in country districts, and not only in poor or primitive countries, but also in the rich nations with an old and highly developed civilisation.[20]

Some historians have stressed the fact that during the interwar period, the American administration considered food as a core of vulnerability in the international order as well as an instrument of influence in foreign policy.[21] Therefore, through the Johns Hopkins School of Public Health, the Rockefeller Foundation and the Experts Committee on Nutrition of the League of Nations, a ledger of global food resources and nutritional requirements was created.[22] National and international organisations recognised a nutrition problem affecting both industrial and agricultural countries even before the 1929 crash. During the early 1930s defective nutrition was not only limited to areas hit by the economic crisis, such as impoverished urban communities and depressed agricultural regions. The awareness of such a situation provoked regional surveys and gave confidence in new scientific concepts as key political tools to overcome the crisis, because "the ill effects of improper feeding are of special gravity in pregnant women and children. Serious and irreparable problems could arise."[23]

During the first decades of the 20th century, scientific research in the field of nutrition led to the search for a scientific formula regarding the *optimum standard of human diet*. As we shall discuss in a further chapter, experimental physiologists identified a total amount of twelve inorganic mineral elements playing an important part in human nutrition. This meant that their absence definitely produced deficiency diseases. Then, there were the vitamins, which were considered to exert a great deal of influence on health. At least the lack of any of nine of

---

20 *Final Report of the Mixed Committee of the League of Nations on Relation of Nutrition to Health, Agriculture and Economic Policy*, Geneva, League of Nations, 1937.

21 Weindling, 1995.

22 *The Problem of Nutrition. Interim Report of the Mixed Committee on the Problem of Nutrition*. Geneva, Series of League of Nations Publications, 1936. [Technical Report A.12.1936.II.B].

23 *The Problem of Nutrition*, 1936, p. 19.

those inorganic elements was experimentally and clinically associated to definite deficiency diseases, defective nutrition or malnutrition.

Under those circumstances, the big objective was not to attempt to prescribe a single type of diet for all the peoples of Europe, but to promote agricultural production to provide the most efficient food supply, taking into consideration the population's traditional dietary habits. Children's health was considered to be the kernel of the problem of nutrition and therefore education and instruction had to become the main instrument of intervention. Science and medicine claimed authority since "ignorance of the principles and main features of the modern science of nutrition is one of the commonest causes of deficiencies in nutrition."[24]

Social, sanitary and cultural implications focused the work to be done on specific information to health professionals, doctors, hygienists, and public health nurses, as well as on instruction of the general public in schools and associations through pamphlets, propaganda, films, posters, pictures and lectures. At the same time economic and agricultural aspects of the problem revealed the necessity for a policy of nutrition and social welfare at a national level in the frame of international coordination. Indeed, nutrition had become an essential part of public health work. Gradually, under the pressure of circumstances, governments were to adopt measures of protection and assistance in regard to food supply, and legislation on food quality, consumption and food codes.[25] These aspects called, first of all, for action on a national level, but also required international co-operation, something indispensable for the efforts made to improve workers' nutrition to be in harmony with the needs of the world economy.

---

[24] *The Problem of Nutrition*, 1936, p. 20-21.

[25] *The Problem of Nutrition*, 1936, p. 66.

CHAPTER 3

Agriculture Serving a Science of Nutrition

The interwar crisis forced the State to play an important active role in improving the availability of foodstuffs for the lower-income sections of the community. In some countries this was done through unemployment insurance policies, minimum wage laws, old age pensions and other social services that made the income of the working classes more secure against cyclical fluctuations.[1] These were probably early versions of Keynesian economic ideology strongly supported by international experts to maintain social stability. A decline in the average size of the family added to the general rise of national revenues, a further argument to support the redistribution role of the State. Controlling agricultural prices to guarantee the availability of farming produce to all the population was essential to political economics.

In addition to economic and technical factors, consumer education also played an important part in overcoming the crisis, since the *new science of nutrition* had disseminated among an ever – increasing section of the population knowledge on the nutritive values of foods. For those that could afford a liberal diet, an abundance of green vegetables, fruit and milk was considered to be more important and richer as a source of mineral matter than wheat bran and wheat germ. Another example shown by nutritionists of the harmful effects of prejudice and ignorance was the decreased consumption of skimmed milk, not substituted by whole milk as desirable, but by a reduction of total milk consumption to the extent that in certain countries and social groups milk was not considered a foodstuff but a medicine.

Once again, the core question was to determine to what an extent agriculture production had adapted to the changes in the demand. Changes should occur gradually as the newer knowledge of nutrition was disseminated among wider groups of the population, the general income was rising, private diet habits changed and special actions were taken by the states to improve the nutritional conditions of particular groups of the population. There was a direct relationship between changes in consumption habits and changes in the demand, which in turn required

---

[1] Trentmann, 2006.

changes in production and food supply. Two main words were uttered by both experts and economists: adjustment and adaptation.

In attempting to define the effort of adaptation required in the important field of agriculture, the emphasis was placed on two points. First, nutrition policy did not involve a rapid transformation in the existing structure of national agricultural systems, and, second, as nutritional policy moved towards its objective of an adequate diet for all, an increase in the demand for all classes of agricultural products was predicted. The demand for protective foods was expected to rise more than the demand for those chiefly consumed for their high energy value.

But in time of crisis not only the population's changing habits and energy requirements were the main concerns. Clearly, the first aim of nutrition policy was to ensure that all sections of the population could afford a sufficient amount of calories. The main tendencies observed suggested that for a long time to come, taking the world as a whole, the increase in the demand for energy-bearing foods among populations suffering from malnutrition would counterbalance the fall in the demand for cereals. It was clear, therefore, that nutrition policy by no means required a drastic shift from the production of energy-bearing foods to the production of protective foods, nor did it require that agriculture should produce protective foods in advance of the market.[2]

Agricultural adaptation was essential to facing the complex situation of nutrition, health and the economy, but important obstacles had to be removed for agriculture to be adapted to the new consumption trends and demands. Special attention had to be paid to the importance of natural conditions and agricultural productive systems in each country. A great deal of capital was needed and the international financial situation was not optimistic at all. On the other hand, culture and tradition played a central role in dietary habits, which appeared to be a factor of deep concern to reach the hard target of adapting production and habits to scientific patterns. More pragmatic obstacles are to be mentioned too: a low level of agricultural technique and the lack of an efficient transport system for commercial networks, since the perishability of certain protective foods made it difficult to ensure availability to all potential consumers. Most of these problems foresaw the further advance of trade globalisation.

During the post 1929 crisis, some national and international agencies certainly made attempts to overcome some big obstacles and so assist agriculture in its task of adaptation. Now and again governmental policy and state social programmes became very important, since changes in

---

2 *Final report*, 1937, p. 160-163.

production, the evolution of agricultural prices, strategies to control production and prices, and the links between income and nutrition habits were crucial aspects of the problem.[3]

Two Conferences of Experts convened in 1932 to discuss nutrition problems during the crisis. The first one – on dietary standards – took place in Rome; the second one, in Berlin, to discuss physical standards and clinical and physiological methods to detect malnutrition.[4] Since nutrition had become a basic part of public health, governments adopted measures of protection and assistance with regard to food supplies. In some countries legislation was enacted,[5] since economic depression and agricultural crisis hindered the availability of food, a price reduction policy was recommended. The prosperity of farmers, peasants and agricultural workers was considered to be an essential element in any policy intended to improve nutrition. Even agricultural practices had to be adapted to meet the new requirements.

As far as the demand tended to be transferred from energy-producing foods to protective foods, the prices of these two categories were considered not to fail to adjust themselves in the same proportion. This adaptation had to act, in itself, as an effective regulator of production. In conclusion, the experts found good reasons for believing that the trend of dietary habits, particularly in Western countries, towards a larger consumption of protective foods would coincide with a parallel evolution in agricultural production, which would in all probability benefit the rural populations of the various countries, and might also greatly contribute to a resumption of normal economic relations between the nations.[6]

Since the Mixed Committee included experts representing the LoN, the ILO and the IIA, we might conclude that access to foodstuffs and nutrition was given international priority in policies and relationships in the 1930s. And in its final report, the Mixed Committee presented fifteen preliminary recommendations to the Assembly of the League of Nations in the hope that they would be accepted by governments as a common political orientation. These recommendations encouraged

---

3 *Final report*, 1937, p. 173.

4 "Conference of Experts for the Standardisation of Certain Methods used in making Dietary Studies. Held in Rome on September 2nd and 3rd, 1932," *League of Nations Quarterly Bulletin of the Health Organisation*, 1932, Vol. 1, No. 1, p. 477-483; "The Most Suitable Methods of Detecting Malnutrition due to the Economic Depression, The. Conference held at Berlin from December 5th to 7th, 1932," *League of Nations Quarterly Bulletin of the Health Organisation*, 1933, Vol. 1, p. 116-129.

5 "Report on the Physiological Bases," 1936, p. 66.

6 "Report on the Physiological Bases," 1936, p. 95.

further scientific research on nutrition problems with a view to ascertaining optimum standards for each country, emphasised the importance of updated information in the teaching of medical students, practitioners, officers and district nurses, following a vigorous policy of education for the general public.

The Mixed Committee showed concern about what steps should be taken to meet the nutritional needs of the lower-income sections of the community – children and the unemployed – to ensure an adequate food supply, especially of protective foods at prices within the reach of all classes. This safeguarded the interests of producers and improved and reduced the cost of marketing and distribution of foodstuffs both in industrial and rural areas, encouraging collaboration between co-operatives and other forms of producers' and consumers' organisations. An international food policy also implied the international unification of the technical analysis and control of foodstuffs, setting up standards of reference and specifications for grading foods of all kinds according to quality. A coordination of the work of different authorities affecting nutrition and food control was recommended as well as the collection of consumption by families of different occupational groups at different income-levels to verify how far national dietaries fell short of the new standards. The committee argued that national statistics on food supply and consumption should be improved and that the International Institute of Agriculture should collect information regarding supply, national consumption and prices.[7]

The mixed committee also offered a survey on the post-war nutritional situation in Europe, South Africa, Australia, Siam and Turkey including measures to improve nutrition in various sections of the population, such as mothers and infants, school-age children and young people, adults, unemployed, and in army and navy dietaries. They suggested measures to reduce prices and make available to consumers foodstuffs at reduced prices, and measures for ensuring the quality of foodstuffs, research, education and popular instruction.

The IIA in Rome contributed fundamental materials, provided information on foodstuffs consumption, as well as on trends in production, prices and consumption, particularly of milk and fresh vegetables in large cities. The international programme also collected data on financial aspects of assistance to national agriculture in various countries, and studied wholesale and retail prices, particularly of protective foods,

7 "Report on the Physiological Bases," 1936, p. 97-98.

relating prices to trends in production and consumption in different countries.[8]

The enormous differences in the diet of western countries were not considered to be accidental but a consequence of local traditions and the changing structure of the labour system. A main tendency was the reduced use of muscular energy as a result of increased mechanisation in industry and agriculture, and a reduction in the hours worked. During the interwar period, an ever smaller fraction of the population was engaged in primary industries of agriculture and forestry. Many people in the countryside were left with no job and an ever-increasing proportion were emigrating to the cities and participated in manufacturing, trade, transportation and professional occupations.[9]

Improvements in housing were considered a way to reduce the amount of food required to keep the body at a constant temperature. The use of automobiles and rapid transport reducing the amount of walking meant that less energy would be spent. Changes in the nature of work and life in modern societies had resulted in changes in food requirements.

Nevertheless, the foods in diets tended to be more expensive than those they had displaced and the state had an important role to play in improving the availability of foodstuffs for lower-income sections of the community through unemployment insurance, minimum wage laws, old age pensions and other social services that secured the working classes' income against cyclical fluctuations. Under those circumstances, rural areas were critical and agricultural prices and product availability to the population reached particular importance.[10]

In addition to economic and technical factors, consumer education played an important part, since the *new science of nutrition* had spread knowledge of the nutritive values of foodstuffs among a constantly increasing section of the population. The idea that governments should get involved in education campaigns both for professionals (doctors, nurses, and teachers) and for the general population was a central argument in most of the experts' reports.[11]

Obviously, during the Depression years, European agriculture had to adapt to new realities. As general incomes rose, special actions would have to be taken to improve the nutrition of particular groups of the

---

8 *Nutrition in various countries*, 1936, p. 269.

9 *Nutrition in various countries*, 1936, p. 267-270.

10 *Final report*, 1937.

11 "Report on the Physiological Bases," 1936; *The Problem of Nutrition*, 1936; *Final Report*, 1937; [McDougall, E.J.] "Rural dietaries," 1939.

community. Changes in consumption habits implied changes in the demand and required transformations in production and food supply. This meant adjustment and adaptation. It was thought that the demand for protective foods was likely to grow more than the demand for those chiefly consumed for their high energy value. In attempting to define the effort of adaptation required of agriculture, particular attention was paid to two points: nutrition policy should not involve a rapid transformation in the existing structure of national agricultural systems, and, as nutritional policy moved towards its objective of an adequate diet for all, an increase in the demand for all classes of agricultural products was expected.[12]

The prosperity of farmers, peasants and agricultural workers was therefore considered an essential element in policies directed towards improved nutrition, but agricultural practice should be adapted to meet the new requirements of better nutrition.[13] Considering the negative effects of the Depression and the agricultural crisis on the nutritional state of the population, one important method of making food available at reduced prices was that of reducing the services provided by the distributor and considering the positive influence, in this field of action, exercised by producers' and consumers' co-operatives. In many countries, these organisations achieved considerable success in their endeavours to reduce the cost of goods to the consumer.[14]

From the political perspective, improved nutrition had to yield immediately general benefits to agriculture and fishing. Better nutrition implied an increase in the demand for foodstuffs, which meant greater agricultural activity. Certain adjustments in agricultural production would be certainly required; adjustments are always needed whenever social change occurs, but their magnitude should be under control, and this meant that the change of habits had to be steady and gradual. Better feeding should contribute immediate benefits to the economy: "While national agricultural systems will thus benefit by the growth in the demand particularly for the more perishable protective foods, countries producing for export will benefit, as the primary needs of the poorer classes for energy-producing and less perishable protective foods are more adequately satisfied."[15] Adaptation in industry, commerce or agriculture also required financial support by national and international agencies and the stimulus of agricultural co-operation. The State had an

12 *Final report*, 1937.
13 *The Problem of Nutrition*, 1936, p. 84.
14 *The Problem of Nutrition*, 1936, p. 83.
15 *Final report*, 1937, p. 45.

important role to play facilitating or impeding the adaptation of agriculture to changes and so the problem of nutrition suddenly became a matter of State.

Under those circumstances tensions between economical agents, states and experts were to appear. While each country was absolutely free and autonomous to decide on its own commercial interests and policies, experts and international agencies claimed for one basic principle the universal acceptance of which was urged, namely, that adequate nutrition was the main factor determining any policies.[16] Due to its worldwide dimension, the problem of nutrition required international collaboration, consultation through national nutrition committees or institutes and international agencies. From an international perspective "the malnutrition which exists in all countries is at once a challenge and an opportunity: a challenge to men's consciences and an opportunity to eradicate a social evil by methods which will increase economic prosperity."[17]

Mixed committees including representatives of the League of Nations, International Labour Office and the International Institute of Agriculture gave nutrition policies priority during the 1930s. They presented recommendations to the governments encouraging further scientific research with a view to ascertaining the optimum standards for each individual country, emphasising the importance of updating information in the teaching of medical students, practitioners, officers, district nurses, following a vigorous policy of education for the general public. The experts required support not only for scientific research but also in promoting the application of modern nutritional science to social practices for the benefit of the different age and occupational groups of the population, as well as facilitating international cooperation in that field. Fighting malnutrition had to become an international commitment led by the League of Nations.[18]

---

16 *Final report*, 1937, p. 50.

17 *Final report*, 1937, p. 53.

18 *Final report*, 1937, p. 54-56.

CHAPTER 4

Guiding Principles for Scientific Studies on Nutrition

The diversity of surveys, reports and features aiming to assess the nutritional state of the European population contributed a big amount of information available for experts and authorities. Unfortunately, most of the work carried out in different countries and the findings presented in international conferences and meetings of experts were not suitable for comparison because of a lack of methodological agreement.

Establishing *physical standards*

Physical standards was the technical name given to anthropometric, clinical and physiological methods used to assess the population's nutritional state. They were employed to identify, from a given group, those suffering from nutritional deficiencies or malnutrition and considered to be in need of dietary treatment. Experimental research on nutrition during the interwar period required the assistance of some systematic clinical screening to be able to assess the effect of dietary regimes on human beings. The problems of establishing satisfactory dietary and physical standards were intimately interconnected, since the ultimate proof of a satisfactory diet was its positive effect on the organism and on health status.[1]

The complexity of factors intervening in human dietary systems and organic nutrition soon gave way to a methodological problem: in attempting to establish standards for an adequate diet, no two physiologists would be likely to reach the same conclusions. A general agreement had not been reached either on the boundaries of *malnutrition* or the methods to identify it in individuals under scientific scrutiny. Physical standards were applied to fulfil several purposes. Parents and family physicians used them to determine children's normal development, and school medical officers requested simple working methods that could be

1 Burnet, Aykroyd, 1935, p. 336.

applied to large groups of children to enable them to spot those suffering from weakness, retarded development and malnutrition.[2]

According to George Newman, since nutrition is connected to the total well-being and right functioning of the whole body a clinical assessment seemed to be necessary.[3] Consequently it should be directly linked to the right functioning of every tissue, organ or system of the body. From a scientific perspective, every aspect of human physiology had to be taken into account to determine the *global state of nutrition* of an individual. Several factors could adversely influence health too, such as the lack of sleep, too much work or hard physical activity, chronic infectious diseases, etc. Some national authorities, such as the British Ministry of Health, assumed those arguments and got engaged in the evaluation of the population's nutritional state.[4]

However, the expression *nutritional status* also included different and more restricted meanings at the time referred to the amount of flesh covering the skeleton. The equivalent of the German term *Ernährungszustand*, this perspective was adopted by some Anglo-American experts. Generally speaking, three different methods of assessing the state of nutrition were mentioned. One was the comparison of certain measures to a standard; another one was the assessment of the state of health and development based on clinical screening; and the last one was a more refined clinical test to detect physiological problems and early deficiency diseases.

Starting with a general check-up, *somatometric* screening aimed to classify the subject according to a type. Height and weight were recorded next to determine an index based on the height-weight-age ratio. Clinical examination was based on the observation of the subject's complexion, mucosae, subcutaneous fat, muscular and nervous systems, bones, teeth, eyes, ears, pharynx, tonsils, lymph glands and sexual primary and secondary characteristics.

Although it was recognised that the height of a child depends on heredity aspects, faulty feeding could influence it if prolonged. Since a child's stature is so variable that single comparisons with standards made no sense, height gain rates and regularity provided useful information, even though growth was not a uniform evolving factor. The various

2 Barona, 2007a, p. 93-96; Perdiguero, E. (ed.), *Salvad al niño. La protección a la infancia en los países de la Europa mediterránea*, Valencia, Seminari d'Estudis sobre la Ciencia, Universitat de València, 2005.

3 Burnet, Aykroyd, 1935, p. 358.

4 *Annual report of the Chief Medical Officer of the Ministry of Health for the year 1933*, Geneva, League of Nations, 1934.

parts of the body have their phases of growth at different times in the course of organic development.[5]

Comparing weight to standards was considered to be of little value, but the weight gain rate and the height-weight ratio were often used in assessing the nutritional status. The so-called *indices of nutrition* were formulated establishing more complicated relationships between height, weight and other bodily measurements, although, concerning children, some experts preferred a simple comparison between the individual's weight and the average height for an age.

Medical experts generally agreed that the most suitable method of assessing nutritional status was clinical examination when done by an experienced physician. Nevertheless, a clinical eye was not compatible with quantitative methods and experimental mentality, and was also criticised for not being reliable enough in the identification of children not clearly undernourished but on the borders between unacceptable nutrition and light deficiencies. Four diagnostic elements were graded: complexion, fat, water content in tissues, and muscle condition. Other methods involved measurements of arm, chest and hip girths.

A great deal of work was devoted to finding out how clinical methods helped to detect children's nutritional status. Obviously, the state of a schoolchild was directly related to his/her health condition; therefore not only physical characteristics were to be studied but also the general functions of the body.[6] To do so, a complete study would require laboratory techniques, not easily available and expensive to run on large groups. Some experts proposed *clinical methods* only, including careful examination of external features, a series of body measurements – the so-called, anthropometry – and the general examination of organs and systems.

The most usual body measurements were height, weight and chest, and sometimes lower and upper limbs. They were compared to average values for a given age or sex, thus providing the *ratio of weight to height*; *ratio of chest measurement to height*, etc. *Pignet's coefficient* (height minus weight plus chest measurement), *Manouvrier's ratio* and other indices were sometimes used.

Since malnutrition caused many organic functions to be impaired, the Conference of Experts in Nutrition convened in Berlin in 1932 proposed a number of physiological tests, such as *physical efficiency*

---

5 Burnet, Aykroyd, 1935, p. 360.

6 Nobécourt, P., Vitry, G. P., "Clinical methods for determining the state of nutrition in school children," *League of Nations Quarterly Bulletin of the Health Organisation*, 1936, Vol. 5, No. 3, p. 544-548.

and fatigability. Some were especially devoted to the early detection of vitamin deficiency, although the clearest evidence of a defective diet, a poor nutritional state or malnutrition was deficiency disease. For the identification of malnutrition, all methods – anthropometric, clinical and physiological – complemented each other. One of the methods recommended by the Berlin Conference, *Pirquet's system*, proved useful in Vienna after the war, but failed in America.

In 1937 a report summarizing the work of the group of experts of the League of Nations appointed to study nutrition evaluation methods in infants and adolescents came to the following general conclusions:[7]

> Methods of assessing the state of nutrition are never simple when the object in view is a specific characterisation of this state in so far as it is clearly related to defective diet.
>
> [...] The comparatively simple, purely somatometric methods that can be used in large-scale enquiries give an indication of the general physical condition of the subject, and the findings do not relate exclusively to the state of nutrition. Anthropological factors connected with differences of stature have an important influence upon the recorded numerical values. The only conditions in which these figures may be of some value in assessing the state of nutrition have been defined.[8]

E.J. Bigwood guiding principles

In order to solve the crucial problem of establishing guidelines to make comparable the diversity of surveys, reports and features aiming to assess the nutritional state of the European population, the experts committee on nutrition of the League of Nations requested E.J. Bigwood, a professor at the University of Brussels, to propose some guiding principles and methods for research. His proposal was presented to the commission of experts in 1938 and the experts agreed on the final wording of Bigwood's *Guide*, to be published shortly after and submitted to the Conference of representatives of the National Nutrition Committees, meeting in October 1938 for its approval.[9] In the meantime, the Secretariat collected data on the state of nutrition of populations living in rural regions of Europe to form preparatory documentation for the 1939 *Rural Life Conference*. Such data were considered to be of great value, particularly when dietary surveys and nutrition assessment

7 "Report on the work of the group of experts appointed to study methods of assessing the state of nutrition in infants and adolescents," *League of Nations Bulletin of the Health Organisation*, 1937, Vol. 6, No. 2, p. 129-204.

8 "Report on the work of the group of experts," 1937, p. 199-200.

9 Bigwood, E.J. *Guiding principles for Studies On the Nutrition of Populations.* Geneva, League of Nations, Technical Commission on Nutrition, 1939.

were combined with information on the general conditions of public health.

Bigwood's monograph responded to a principal aim, i.e. to point out what elements should be born in mind in conducting nutrition surveys of populations so that the work could be carried out and the findings presented in such a way so as to facilitate comparison, a need identified by all experienced workers in this field.[10] Bigwood was aware that, in many cases, records could not be fully exploited because the investigations concerned had not been planned in a manner ensuring comparability and therefore most efforts were not useful. Standardisation of research methods was a challenge to face without interfering with originality of research. His guidelines included a description of methods of studying the physiological problems associated with nutrition suitable for application to population groups of different sizes and diverse physiological, demographic and social characteristics.

The two main aspects to challenge were, on the one hand, dietary surveys and, on the other, enquiries into the state of nutrition of the population. Bigwood proposed four types of dietary surveys: statistical studies of food resources in a country; studies covering particular, more or less homogeneous, social groups and institutions; classification of families into homogeneous and representative groups, and exclusively individual enquiries. Survey methods were detailed: weighing method, records of purchases in special household books, and questionnaires. The scope and duration of surveys, as well as the number and the qualifications of investigators were taken into consideration. A list and classification of foodstuffs designed to facilitate international comparison was also proposed.

Once the surveys had been completed, a physiological analysis of the data obtained had to be undertaken and, therefore, Bigwood discussed the factors to be considered in the study of the physiological value of the diet. He proposed a general classification of essential nutritive principles in the diet, food waste, energy-bearing principles and protective principles, including food composition tables. When discussing the biological value of proteins and chemical elements and vitamins, his monograph summarised nutritional knowledge and tried to propose scales of family consumption coefficients for calories and nutritive principles other than energy-bearing. Nevertheless he recognised the adoption of scales of calories coefficient as the only suitable instrument at the time. In the case of dietary constituents instead of energy-bearing ones, he preferred to make assessments per head, regardless of age or sex. Since different

---

10 Bigwood, 1939, see general introduction.

scales for calories, protective principles and cost of diet had been proposed, Bigwood concluded that, regardless of the system adopted, it was essential to indicate in detail the valued respectively adopted as scale units for the several nutritive principles.

Moreover, an economy perspective was also considered comparing the cost of different foodstuffs in one country and in different areas, the cost of diet and subsequent scales of family coefficients for cost of diet. Statistical considerations were also stressed when talking about dietary surveys, such as the distribution of a phenomenon around the mean, median value and mode, symmetry or asymmetry of dispersion, dispersion index and standard error of the mean.

When discussing the guidelines for the enquiries into the state of nutrition of the population, somatometric tests, clinical tests and physiological tests all came into consideration. Bigwood analysed trends of the mean weight and mean height of groups of children as well as various somatometric indices. Measurement of the thickness of the skin and of the immediately subjacent tissues; determination of the state of development of the muscles, examination of the teeth, the sign of the dorsal median furrow took part of the clinical tests proposed. Bigwood finally discussed specific physiological tests to detect malnutrition, vitamin A deficiency, and others to detect early vitamin D and C pre-deficiency as well as pre-deficiencies of organic chemical elements and proteins. He discussed various types of enquiries in a number of countries concluding that the methods available to assess the state of nutrition of the population were never simple when the object in view was a specific characterisation of this state in so far as it was clearly related to a defective diet.

The comparatively simple, purely somatometric methods used in large-scale enquiries gave an indication of the all-round physical condition of the subject, although the results did not exclusively relate to the state of nutrition. Anthropological factors connected with differences of stature had an important influence upon the recorded numerical values. The more complex methods tried to combine simple somatometric tests with either clinical or physiological tests, but they were not suitable at the time for use in large-scale enquiries. More detailed investigations were expected to yield new knowledge concerning scales of states of malnutrition, but they were in the experimental stage. Therefore, Bigwood recommended combining, wherever possible, dietary surveys and enquiries into the state of nutrition, covering the same population groups. His proposals were accepted by the League of Nations and served as international references.

CHAPTER 5

Food and Nutrition in Various Countries

The landscape in the early 1920s

The critical situation of the food supply and the poor nutritional condition of Europe's population dated back to the Great War years, becoming a chronic problem in the 1920s. The high cost of food in Europe cast a very dark shadow and, according to the specialists, chronic hunger threatened Europe's health.[1] In a paper published in 1922, the Catalan physiologist August Pi i Sunyer compared the prices of basic foodstuffs in Berlin, Barcelona and other European cities and concluded that European people were much poorer in 1922 than in 1914. Making a comparison between the average income and food prices, Pi i Sunyer determined the threshold of poverty, identifying it in those sectors of the population that had to spend 70% of their income on food. He estimated that in 1922 in Barcelona "reducing the food expenditure under 1.75 pesetas per person per day is certainly the way towards insufficient nutrition..."[2] Early in the 1920s, the victims of poor nutrition were counted by millions in Russia, China, Germany, Austria, the Balkan countries and Poland, and in Spain, regions like the *Hurdes* showed the ravages of poverty on health and physical development in many populations, especially those living in the countryside in a situation of semi-exclusion.[3] The social and medical perception that a deep crisis resulted from a poor diet alarmed politicians and put European states into action.

The effects of depression

Laboratory and clinical research available in the early 1930s made it clear that the health of a nation was closely bound up with the state of nutrition of its population. It seemed therefore important to discover what kind of food the unemployed millions, with an income reduced to a

1 Pi i Sunyer, A., *El hambre de los pueblos*, Conferencia dada en la Academia de Medicina en 29 de enero de 1922, Barcelona, Asociación instructiva de obreros y empleados municipales, 1922.

2 Pi i Sunyer, 1922, p. 23.

3 *Viaje a las Hurdes. El manuscrito inédito de Gregorio Marañón y las fotografías de la visita de Alfonso XIII*, Madrid, El País-Aguilar, 1993.

very low level, were able to buy as a consequence of the international crisis. While very few studies of the dietaries actually used by unemployed men and their families had been made during previous years, sufficient data existed to enable certain inferences about nutrition in lower income groups.[4] Specialists in the new experimental physiology of nutrition adapted calorie requirements to the new critical situation.

A sedentary worker was supposed to need from 2,200 to 2,400 calories a day. This was estimated by subtracting from the 3,100 calories needed by an average worker the 800 calories demanded by an average day's work. Therefore, during the period of unemployment calorie needs could be reduced by 27% for workers and around 8% for the entire family. Based on to figures on food expenditure and income of a number of families of unemployed families collected by the German *Statistisches Reichsamt* some evidence of under-nourishment was shown for 1927, a year of relative prosperity, but the financial position of the unemployed had steadily worsened ever since. A 19% fall in the cost of living and a 25% one in food prices had taken place between 1927 and 1932, the situation being described as a hidden famine.[5] An estimate of the state of nutrition among the unemployed in Germany, which was based entirely on official figures relating to allowances and market prices, slightly over-accentuated the seriousness of the situation, since only 45% of the available income went on food. If unemployed families spent on food this proportion of their income, the number of calories purchasable would be about 532 to 1,140 per day for children and 840 to 1,800 for adults. Some detailed dietaries regarding unemployed families in Germany talked about the difficult situation: in three meals out of four, very little other than coffee and bread with margarine or jam was eaten. The midday meal usually included a greater variety of foodstuffs – soup, potatoes, green vegetables, and sometimes meat.[6]

In Britain technical reports for 1932 showed that the total income of the unemployed just about covered the necessary food expenditure but the safety margin was very small. At the time, the situation in Germany was comparatively worse. Food availability was a central factor from the perspective of both domestic and foreign affairs. Accordingly to the British Ministry of Health "the diet in the households of the unemployed men comprised little beyond white bread, butter or margarine, potatoes,

4 "The Economic Depression and Public Health, Memorandum prepared by the Health Section. III. The Nutrition of the Unemployed," *League of Nations Quarterly Bulletin of the Health Organisation*, 1932, Vol. 1, p. 443-457.

5 "The Economic Depression and Public Health," 1932, p. 448.

6 Report by Lehmann in 1931 included in "The Economic Depression and Public Health," 1932, p. 452.

sugar, jam, tea and bacon in limited quantity: although meat was seldom eaten, fresh milk was not seen and the usual milk was skimmed condensed. Fresh vegetables other than potatoes were seldom eaten.[7]

Such disproportion between the income of the unemployed and their necessary food expenditure existed in many other European countries. General awareness of a loss of quality was inevitably increasing, the resulting tendency being an increased consumption of cheaper vegetable foods at the expense of milk, meat, eggs and butter. This tendency had to be counteracted by mass production to meet an urgent demand for very cheap animal foods.

According to international expert surveys, in the Far East, Tropical Countries and Colonial territories dietary standards were not essentially different from those of Western countries. Further comparative studies of physiological differences due to cultural habits and climate and their possible bearing on food requirements were indeed desirable in those areas. Since a scientific approach was based on the idea that physiological standards were universally applicable, they had to be expressed in terms of the dietary habits of the various peoples.

Research work on nutrition in the Far East prompted the study of the nutritive value of local foodstuffs, the diet of the different population groups, their state of nutrition and the incidence of diseases caused by dietary deficiencies. In order to carry out diet surveys for different population groups, data had to be calculated not only in terms of food factors (calories, nutritional principles, vitamins, minerals, etc.) but also in terms of real foodstuffs consumed, i.e. in terms of diet. Such investigations were expected to contribute a definition of the problem in any case and therefore encourage the consumption of certain products: under-milled rice, red palm oil and others. Feeding experiments on groups were suggested by nutritionists.

The League of Nations' Technical Commission on nutrition underlined the importance of relying on natural local products, but they also agreed that certain population groups could benefit from the distribution of pure and concentrated vitamins, provided these could be obtained cheaply in large quantities. Yeast, a product rich in nitrogenous elements and B group vitamins, was considered to be of particular value in correcting deficiencies in the diets of tropical and Eastern populations. Something similar was said about mineral elements, which could be supplied cheaply to schoolchildren and groups suffering from a deficiency of these elements. One of the most important defects of the so-

---

7 "The Economic Depression and Public Health," 1932, p. 452.

called *poor rice-eater's diet* – a problem identified in some Asian regions – was precisely calcium shortage.

Raising education standards and giving specific instruction on the principles of nutrition was considered necessary for all social classes and as an instrument to improve dietary habits in each country.

In 1938 circumstances were very critical in Europe. For two years Spain suffered the shortages derived from the civil war and a severe restriction of foodstuffs aggravated the nutrition problem in many other European countries to the extent that emergency measures by governments against famine as a real threat were needed. National institutes of food had been created in most countries to coordinate food policy, trade and availability. Under those circumstances, the League of Nations' Technical Commission on Nutrition took on the task of implementing a dietary standard trying to ensure an optimum degree of nutrition. On the other hand, the approach to famine relief was largely dependent on local circumstances. In this regard, important factors had to be taken into account such as the relation between available funding and the numbers to be fed, food transport and storage, fuel supply, etc. As a consequence, several programmes to prevent famine were proposed by the Technical Commission.

The evolution of the work done by the Technical Commission and its field of implementation took a shift at the end of the 1930s, from a scenario in which *optimum diet* was the aim in a wide project implying agriculture, health, experimental research and politics, to quite a different one threatened by malnutrition and famine.

CHAPTER 6

Experts in Action: Physiology of Nutrition and Optimum Diet

From a purely physiological rationality, the principles of correct nutrition stated that the diet had to supply the necessary substances for the growth and repair of the organism, as well as energy for the production of animal heat and muscular work. Experimental science was to be the necessary basis of any practical action.[1] Experiments with animals seemed to be useful to clarify fundamental aspects of human nutrition, but only the screening of humans and the analysis of clinical data could contribute to establishing standards.

Dietary standards and the nutritive value of food

Scientifically speaking, the fundamental principles of the new science of nutrition were not as firmly established as they were in other experimental sciences. Many accepted facts were debatable and laws which seemed fully established years before were opened to question as a consequence of further research. Physiology of nutrition was still a body of knowledge in progress. Since living organisms were not to be considered to behave only as thermodynamic machines – because organisms tend to adapt to changes in their environment and dietary habits – the problems of energy and protein requirements were still being discussed. There were so many variable factors operating that the interpretation of dietary experiments was extremely difficult. Moreover, animal experiments were insufficient to clarify all aspects of human nutrition. As shown in previous pages, in the international conferences held in the 1930s methodological debates and standardised methods of research and measurement opened up new avenues; international agreement on methods and standards was therefore necessary.

There were, however, a number of facts which were firmly established. The organism needed to be supplied daily with a certain quantity of food energy that could be evaluated in terms of calories and, from the beginning of the experimental science of nutrition, a considerable amount of information on calorie requirements was increasingly avail-

[1] Burnet, Aykroyd, 1935, p. 334.

able. It was accepted that food factors such as vitamins and mineral salts were essential to health but, at the same time, it was also clear that they did not affect the fundamental problem of energy needs. The daily diet had to yield protein, fat and carbohydrate, their proportion varying according to circumstances. On the other hand, small amounts of minerals were also considered necessary, the most important being phosphorus, calcium, iron and iodine, as well as vitamins and other essential factors.[2]

However, it was generally admitted that the energy needs of the body were supplied by fats, carbohydrates and proteins, proteins having the additional function of building new tissue for the growing animal and of repairing tissue wastage in the adult.[3] In addition, experimental research on the physiology of nutrition had stressed the great importance of other essential elements, such as vitamins and minerals, which were also deemed indispensable. The lack of those elements or their defective presence in dietaries was related to deficiency diseases and children's organic development.

The new experimental physiology of nutrition aimed to take a step forward in the determination of human dietary standards. Physiologists in previous decades had generally devoted their attention to the establishment of minimum dietary requirements.[4] Such was also the usual standpoint of Governments and administrations when called upon to fix the rations for bodies of workers, or to feed large numbers of soldiers and civilians in wartime, or when obliged to assist the unemployed and their families during the time of industrial depression. Minimum dietary requirements were the keystone. Nevertheless, the idea of an *optimum diet* was developed during the interwar period and brought into preeminence as a more meaningful concept. An optimum diet was one providing for the full development of the individual for efficiency without exhaustion and for his resistance to disease.[5]

Diseases such as scurvy, rickets, beriberi or pellagra were identified as being associated with deficient nutrition. Therefore, according to medical knowledge, nutrition was to become an essential factor to enjoy optimum health, a condition necessary to fight infectious diseases. Since the late 1920s, malnutrition, poverty, children's diseases, and economic crisis paved the road for a new field of action, and the idea of a *standard*

---

2 Burnet, Aykroyd, 1935, p. 323-474.

3 *The Problem of Nutrition*, 1936, p. 32.

4 Livi-Bacci, M., *Population and Nutrition: An Essay on European Demographic History*, Cambridge, Cambridge University Press, 1991.

5 *The Problem of Nutrition*, 1936, p. 53.

for adequate nutrition was widely accepted as a starting point for future policies.[6]

According to the *London Report*, a dietary standard had to take into account energy requirements, the proportion of protective foods, and mineral and vitamin requirements.[7] Once those general aspects were clearly determined, further research was to focus on specific problems such as nutritive requirements during the first year of life and infancy. Since a common methodology was needed in order to allow comparisons, the Technical Commission on Nutrition of the League of Nations shaped some guiding principles for experimental research and social surveys.[8]

The notion of *optimum diet* had been introduced at the beginning of the 20th century, based on physiological research on calorie intake and expenditure, and protein, fat, mineral and vitamin requirements. Foodstuffs were classified into two main groups: *protective foods*, such as milk, eggs, meat, cheese, vegetables, potatoes and cod-liver oil; and *supplementary energy-yielding foods*, such as cereals, fats and sugar. A new *calorific method* was then introduced to calculate individual needs according to tables based on *energetic quotients* so that calorie requirements could be assessed to ensure the healthy development of the human organism. The calorie represented a universal value to measure nutrition across time, nations, ages and races.[9]

The Mixed Technical Commission on nutrition of the League of Nations, International Labour Organisation and International Institute of Agriculture convened in London in November 1935. The Commission told the national academies of medicine and the national commissions competent in nutritional problems to implement those policies. A preliminary "Report on the Physiological Basis of Nutrition" (1936) was published including an interim report with their suggestions.[10] Edward Mellanby presided over the Technical Commission; E. Burnet and W. R. Aykroyd carried out a series of enquiries in different countries (United Kingdom, France, USA, Denmark, Sweden, Norway and the USSR) and R. Cathcart, an expert on quantitative methods in nutrition, chaired the sessions. Members included physiologists, clinicians and statisticians.

---

6 Burnet, Aykroyd, 1935; Caplan, P. (ed.), *Food, Health and Identity*, London, Routledge, 1997.

7 *The Problem of Nutrition*, 1936.

8 Bigwood, E.J., *Guiding Principles for Studies On the Nutrition of Populations. Technical Commission on Nutrition*, Health Organisation of the League of Nations Geneva, 1939. [C.H.1401; C.H./Com.Exp.Alim./50(2)].

9 Bigwood, E.J., *Guiding Principles.*

10 Archive of the League of Nations, Document C.H.1197.

Their main scientific aim was to reach significant findings to obtain a formula for an optimum human diet standard. It was accepted that twelve inorganic mineral elements played an important part in human nutrition and that their absence produced deficiency diseases. In addition, vitamins were a large territory for exploration because of their important influence on health. The absence of any nine of these vitamins caused deficiency diseases or defective nutrition. The pathological effects of improper feeding were particularly serious in pregnant women and children.[11]

Surveys discussed by the Experts' Committee on Nutrition showed that family diets within the same food expenditure group varied widely across Europe. The instruction of doctors and hygienists was a first step, with National Schools of Hygiene playing an important role. In addition, education was to target the general population through school campaigns, pamphlets, propaganda, films, posters and pictures.

In 1936, the International Labour Organisation published a report on "Workers' Nutrition and Social Policy," addressing two main questions. First, "what light do family budget enquiries throw upon the diets of workers in different countries and at different levels of the income scale?"[12] Second, "what approaches have been made by social and labour legislation towards improving the nutrition of workers?"[13] The report concluded with an analysis of the educational, research and socio-economic problems involved in raising levels of nutrition to the desired standards.

The physiology of nutrition stated that the diet had to supply the necessary substances for the growth and repair of the organism and energy for the production of animal heat and muscular work.[14] But nutritional research had also stressed the importance of vitamins and minerals.[15] This perspective allowed a table to be devised containing the nutritive values of foodstuffs. Dietary needs were analysed according to social and age groups and paying special attention to expectant and nursing mothers. With regard to the health of both mother and offspring, protective foodstuffs would have a large effect on eliminating many of the ills of pregnancy.[16]

---

11 "Report on the Physiological Bases," 1936.

12 "Nutrition and Labour. Survey of the Nutrition Problem by the ILO," in *The Problem of Nutrition*, 1936.

13 *The Problem of Nutrition*, 1936, p. 70.

14 "Report on the Physiological Bases," 1936, p. 32.

15 "Report on the Physiological Bases," 1936, p. 32.

16 "Report on the Physiological Bases," 1936, p. 39.

In early childhood, nutrition was considered essential to maintain resistance against infectious diseases. Compulsory education had been generally adopted throughout western countries,[17] but children could not be mentally or physically fit without the right nutrition.[18] In the case of adolescents, young soldiers and adults, although "further enquiries will be necessary to establish the influence of certain given foodstuffs on human susceptibility or resistance to infection, there can be no doubt as to the general value of a proper diet in increasing resistance to disease."[19]

Evidence on vitamin deficiency diseases (scurvy, rickets, beriberi, pellagra) reinforced the scientific project of reaching a universal standard for an optimum and minimum diet. The London Report made room for the concept of *dietary standards* taking into account protective foods, energy, mineral and vitamin requirements, and their proportion in milk, eggs, meat, green and leafy vegetables, fruits, cod-liver oil and energy-bearing foods. During the first eight months of life, breastfeeding and later artificial feeding supplemented with vitamin-rich substances were strongly recommended. To prevent anaemia, egg yolk, purees of green vegetables or carrots, and iron salts were also prescribed. In the case of premature infants, further supplementary vitamins and minerals were to be added.

As we have already discussed in a previous chapter, it seemed impossible to define precisely the normal standards of health and physical development in order to set the boundaries of the pathological. Empirical research and clinical data showed that there existed border-line conditions between health and pathology which were hard to detect and define. During the interwar period, methods to assess nutritional status were questioned from a scientific point of view, although they were useful for practical action. The same applied to discussions about the validity of the so-called *indices of nutrition*, introduced for clinical purposes in the measurement of height, weight, chest width, hip and arm girth and other anthropometric data. They were mainly applied to chil-

---

17 Although national regulations differed from one country to the other, a common element was the responsibility of the state and its regulatory task. See Hendrick, H., *Child Welfare. Historical Dimension, Contemporary Debate*, Cambridge, Polity Press, 2003. In the case of Spain, compulsory education until 12 years of age was regulated in 1901. Nevertheless, most children left school before this age, especially in rural areas. See Barona, J. L., Cherry S., *Health and Medicine in Rural Europe (1850-1945)*, Valencia, Seminari d'Estudis sobre la Ciència, Universitat de València, 2005.

18 "Report on the Physiological Bases," 1936, p. 48.

19 "Report on the Physiological Bases," 1936, p. 53.

dren and used to determine underdevelopment, insufficient nutrition and those pre-clinical states conceptualised as *weakness* and *consumption.*

The League of Nations' Technical Commission on Nutrition submitted a report to the Health Committee in April-May 1936 and to the General Council in May 1936. The Health Committee suggested further work to attain practical effects in different countries, with specific research on food requirements during the first year of life and the implementation of social policies to scientifically assess the nutritional state of children, pregnant women, workers, and ideally the whole population.[20] Technical aspects of research had to be covered and conceptual agreements reached, such as coefficients for calculating calories and proteins according to age and sex, particularly as regards maternity, infancy and periods of organic growth and convalescence. Special requirements during certain periods of life characterised by strong change like puberty were also discussed, as well as the official control of fish-liver oil and vitamin preparations.

The observations sent by national boards were studied by the Technical Commission in its 2nd session held in Geneva on 4-8 June, 1936.[21] The main points on the agenda consisted of a critical review of the *London Report* on the physiological bases of nutrition to oversee the progress of studies on the problems recommended in it, followed by some specific topics, such as milk consumption, the physiological properties of milk and research on nutrition in Chile. The second part of the Conference was focused on the assessment of children's nutritional condition and the means to prevent, identify, and cure malnutrition. The main difficulties emerged from the necessity to establish fixed standards for the optimum diet. Since health and nutrition are closely related, a distinction could be made between primary malnutrition due to a defective diet and secondary malnutrition resulting from illness. The technical commission insisted on the fact that vitamin and mineral deficiency showed specific clinical signs and symptoms that could indeed be detected. It implied improving clinical examination methods would be able to identify all relevant signs.

The following working session of the Technical Commission took place at the beginning of 1937. Two main topics drew attention, the first one was related to energy, protein and fat requirements associated with calorie production and consumption in the light of the influence of

---

20 "Report on the Physiological Bases," 1936, p. 391-415.

21 "Report by the Technical Commission on Nutrition on the work of its second session held in Geneva, June 4th to 8th, 1936," *League of Nations Quarterly Bulletin of the Health Organisation*, 1936, Vol. 5, No. 3, p. 416-426.

climate on dietary requirements, and the second one focused on mineral and vitamin requirements. Physiological conditions such as pregnancy and lactation, and age groups – childhood and adulthood – were specifically discussed.

The general principle of a good diet was repeated: people had to be made aware of the healthy effects of a varied diet; variety in diet leads to safety, provided it contains sufficient protective foodstuffs. The Commission warned about the increasing use of white flour, deprived of important nutritive elements. Its use was to be cut down and partially substituted by milled cereals and potatoes. They also alerted experts to the excessive consumption of sugar.

In March 1937, the Technical Commission on Nutrition of the League of Nations was composed of sixteen members, E. Mellanby being its President. Some specific commissions for technical studies were integrated by national representatives.[22] The Spanish representation was entrusted to the *Real Academia de Medicina de Madrid*.[23]

According to the Commission, children had to be systematically examined to determine their nutritional status. Malnutrition being a complex category, efforts had to be made to devise appropriate tests. Wide discussions on somatometric indices took place. A more specific topic that drew the Commission's attention was that of nutritional requirements in the first year of life. Once more, breastfeeding was strongly recommended during the first eight or nine months of the infant. When this was not possible, the recommended diet was milk supplemented by substances rich in vitamins A, C and D in order to prevent the risk of anaemia: "… the addition to the diet of all infants of small amounts of food rich in iron is advocated from an early age."[24] Premature infants were considered a special group needing a greater amount of supplementary vitamins and mineral additions to the diet. The practice of giving cereal foods before the sixth month of life was not advised; after this, potatoes were recommended as partial substitutes for cereals as well as full-fat milk.

Experimental studies on milk composition in animals offered valuable information about its content of nitrogen and calcium salts, positive elements for growth and the prevention of dental disease. Reports on the

---

22 League of Nations, Health General, R.6133, Registry No. 8A, 21287, 20883. 1933-1939. Nutrition. Technical Commission on Nutrition. Reports, printing. Archives of the League of Nations.

23 It consisted of three members: Teófilo Hernando, E. Suñer and J. Murillo, director of the Institute for the Control of Food and Medicines.

24 *Health Organisation Report*, Geneva, League of Nations, 1936, p. 6.

minimum amount of milk, potatoes and cereals were also discussed, as well as research in elementary schools on the influence of adding supplementary milk to children's diet. Similar studies were devoted to pregnant women. Since those experimental investigations seemed to be very important for the future, the technical commission also suggested recourse to the national institutions, academies and research councils to stimulate research.[25] The impact of the London report was so intense that it was discussed in most of the League of Nations meetings held in following years.[26]

What constitutes a balanced diet? Answering this general question meant specifying the human requirements of calories, fat, proteins, vitamins and minerals, and establishing the right proportions in which the various nutritional factors had to be combined. The nutritive value of food was to be the basis for dietary standards. And again, by what means could the nutritional state of an individual be assessed and how could malnutrition get screened? Dietary standards were the starting point for further practical action; they allowed experts to gauge the value of the diet of individuals or social groups, making it possible to draw up dietary schedules for those communities or social groups that had no choice, like armies, inmates at institutions, schoolchildren, and prisoners. They were also used as the basis of large-scale wartime rationing schemes and as a starting point for future agricultural policies.

Human calorie requirements were investigated by direct and indirect calorimetric methods to determine the energy output of subjects at rest or performing various kinds of work. Experimental conditions provided data for the establishment of quantitative standards of food intake. Another method consisted of assessing dietary requirements by means of the observation of what healthy individuals living under various conditions and performing different kinds of works consumed.

The basal metabolic rate of an average European citizen was considered to range from 65 to 75 calories per hour, the energy exchange being lower during sleep and considerably higher during physical activities. The increase in energy exchange in relation to the basal metabolism, which takes place during the performance of different activities, was carefully investigated in the laboratory. As a result, it was possible to put together an energy budget for an average individual during an average day, which was found to be about 3,000 calories per day. This

25 One of the first reports referred to Norway: "Appreciation de l'état de nutrition des enfants. Remarques préliminaires Dr. C. Schiötz (Oslo), 25.2.1936."

26 It was a main topic of debate at the League of Nations, Health General, R. 6134, Registry No. 8A, 23831, 20883. Une Conférence juin 1936, Genève.

figure was widely used in practical dietetics, put forward as a standard by the Advisory Committee on Nutrition of the British Ministry of Health, and accepted by V. Tyzska, one of the most influential German specialists.

A crucial point was the acknowledgment that energy requirements varied enormously according to the type of work performed, from about 6,000 or 7,000 calories in the case of a lumberman to 2,200 for a sedentary worker.[27] The energy requirements of children and women were considered to be lower than those of an adult man. Both statistical and calorimetric data regarding calorific intake and requirements were registered for both sexes and age groups as the basis of *scales of family coefficients*, which calculated the needs of children and women in terms of an average man, the latter being taken as the standard. More than twenty different scales of family coefficients were proposed. Most of them estimated the energy requirements of women to be about 0.8 of those of an adult man, something acceptable for industrial areas but hardly representative of reality in peasant communities, where housewives worked at home and side by side with their husbands in the fields.

Such scales allowed the establishment of a *consumption unit* in terms of which the requirements of the entire group could be calculated. The scales of family coefficients were essential to finding out family dietary habits, comparing the total food intake with other families. The total food intake of each family was divided by the number of consumption units, usually estimated as the need of an adult man. Nevertheless, some authors questioned previous knowledge about certain aspects such as the relationship between calorie intake and physical effort.[28]

The Conference of Experts for the Standardisation of Certain Methods used in making Dietary Studies convened in Rome on September 2nd and 3rd, 1932 some years before Bigwood guidelines were published.[29] The agenda of the Conference included reaching an international agreement on a scale or scales of family coefficients, *family consumption units*, an excellent instrument of analysis in making dietary studies, in order to make the results comparable. Although this was the main target of the Conference, other questions were also discussed:

[27] Burnet, Aykroyd, 1935, p. 339.

[28] Bigwood, E.J., Roost, G., *L'alimentation rationnelle et les besoins énergétiques d'une population ouvrière*, Bruxelles, Université Libre de Bruxelles, Institut Solvay, 1934, 256 p.

[29] "Conference of Experts for the Standardisation of Certain Methods used in making Dietary Studies. Held in Rome on September 2nd and 3rd, 1932," *League of Nations Quarterly Bulletin of the Health Organisation*, 1932, Vol. 1, No. 1, p. 477-483.

a) Accuracy and uniformity of food values used in the assessment of data to determine the factors to be studied.

b) Common principles with regard to the techniques employed in investigating the dietary habits of population groups.

c) Definitions of the terms *light*, *moderate* and *severe* work, as well as *average day's manual work* in terms of kilograms.

In order to facilitate the comparison of dietary enquiries conducted in different countries, it seemed advantageous to have an internationally agreed scale of "family coefficients," but the existing scientific data were not sufficient to allow the construction of a scale corresponding to real values.

The Conference argued that no scale could be formulated reflecting the food consumption of families in all countries and in all circumstances of life. The variation, from country to country and from class to class, of such factors as height, weight, etc. made it impossible for one particular scale to match real values everywhere. It was therefore agreed that, in putting forward an international scale, no pretence of absolute accuracy could be made. The international scale should be of a comparatively uncomplicated nature, i.e. the coefficients chosen should be simple fractions, according to age and sex comparatively limited. Two objections were made to putting forward a highly detailed scale. First, statistical offices and nutritional research workers might be reluctant to use it; second, it could convey a false appearance of accuracy. Subject to these hypotheses, the scale chosen for an international use had to correspond as closely as possible with the scientific data available.

The Expert Committee on Nutrition convened by the League of Nations in 1932 produced the following scale, being 1 a calculated amount of 3,000 calories:[30]

Age	Male	Coefficient both sexes	Female
0-2		0.2	
2-3		0.3	
4-5		0.4	
6-7		0.5	
8-9		0.6	
10-11		0.7	
12-13		0.8	
14-59	1.0		0.8
Over 60		0.8	

30 *League of Nations Quarterly Bulletin of the Health Organisation*, Vol. 1, (1932), p. 480.

Though it was not a perfect scale, this international proposal was widely employed to make results easily comparable. The Rome Conference also suggested that researchers engaged in dietary enquiries should, if possible, provide information, not only with regard to the intake of calories, protein, carbohydrate, and fat, but also with regard to the intake of animal or vegetable protein.

The members of the technical commission taking part in the Conference concluded that it was impossible, based on the knowledge they had, to put forward a useful definition of the terms *light*, *moderate* and *severe* work, or of an *average day's manual work*, given the large differences across countries and regions. In any case, the principles of adequate nutrition were based on a well balanced diet.

The first serious attempt to set up a dietary standard was made by Carl von Voit in his book *Food and the Principles of Dietetics* (London, 1927). Using a calorimeter, he calculated that a man weighing about 70 kilograms and doing moderate work needs daily 3,055 calories, 118 grams protein, 58 grams fat and 500 grams carbohydrates. Other standards proposed by experts on physiology of nutrition, such as Atwater, Rubner and Hutchinson, did not differ significantly.[31]

Protein requirements

Heated discussions on the optimum protein intake among physiologists, physicians, economists and other professionals with an interest in nutrition took place during the 1930s. Even among experimental scientists, some advocated a high intake while others emphasised restricted consumption. To a certain extent, contradictory clinical evidence about the effects of high protein diets on the kidneys contributed to the debate. Some experiments had shown that diets containing 30% of protein produced signs of kidney damage in rabbits and human beings, but those results had been criticised alleging that experimental diets were incomplete regarding dietary components other than protein. Other experiments showed that hypertrophy and congestion of the kidneys occurred in rats fed on diets containing 30 to 40% of protein but containing a balanced proportion of vitamins and minerals. In spite of kidney damage, the animals were in excellent general condition. On the contrary, rats seemed to be in perfect health in other experiments after one year on a diet containing 70% protein. In most of such experiments, the proportion of protein in the diet greatly exceeded that in the ordinary, freely-

31 Aykroyd, W.R., "Diet in relation to small incomes," *League of Nations Quarterly Bulletin of the Health Organisation*, 1933, Vol. 1, p. 130-153.

chosen diets of Western societies.[32] Physiologists, on the whole, agreed on the fact that societies with a high protein intake have a better organic development than those with a lower one, but no inference could be drawn as to the optimum protein consumption.

In support of a low intake, many population groups consuming less than 70 grams of protein per day in rural areas of Europe were described as healthy, although little was known about their vital statistics, resistance to disease or even their physical potentialities with a richer diet. Under those uncertain circumstances, the minimum amount of protein required to ensure nitrogenous metabolism was investigated. Some experiments claimed that health and nitrogenous balance could be maintained on a diet of cereals, potatoes, margarine and fruit containing only 32 grams of absorbable protein. This was the lowest level put forward. One of the specialists at the Laboratory for Nutrition Research in Copenhagen, M. Hindhede, proposed a protein standard of 60 grams, combined with a calorie standard of 2,500.[33] But he was criticised for being a follower of the "return to nature," and his view was controversial in the economic sphere, since he considered it a big mistake to transform cheap food into expensive food by feeding pigs on cereals which could with advantage be fed directly to human beings; he also urged the consumption of non milled cereals. Laboratory experiments suggested that a sustained diet with a very low protein content produced weakness, although it was admitted that other factors could also be involved. Between two such protein extremes – a very high one and a very low one – it was difficult to prove experimentally that one level of intake was preferable to the other. It was not convenient to adopt – as a standard – the lowest amount of protein to which the body could adjust, therefore 1 gram of protein per kilo of body-weight or about 70 grams for an average man was considered to be a suitable standard. But the authority of other specialists finally led to the general acceptance of a *protein standard* of 100 grams in Europe and a bit lower in America.

It was usually assumed that some of the protein contained in a satisfactory diet had to be of animal origin, as it was thought to have a higher biological value than vegetable protein. The Advisory Committee on Nutrition of the British Ministry of Health has suggested 37 grams as a suitable daily allowance of "first class" or animal protein for an average

32 Burnet, Aykroyd, 1935, p. 342-343.

33 Hindende, M., "The Effect of Food Restriction During War on Mortality in Copenhagen," *Journal of the American Medical Association*, 1920, Vol. 74, No. 6.

man, which would represent about 5% of total calories on a diet yielding 3,000 calories per day.[34]

During growth, protein and mineral requirements are obviously relatively greater than in adult life. For practical public health work, a standard from 70 to 100 grams of proteins was employed, a reasonable share being of animal origin even though the tendency of dietary prescriptions in many European countries pointed to a decrease in meat consumption. A report on protein needs and consumption carried out by E.F. Terroine (1936) offered some general conclusions.[35] Whenever proteins are present in the diet in quantities exceeding those which are necessary to meet the specific nitrogenous needs of the body, and are used as energy-bearing foods, this was both a physiological and economic malpractice. In every rationally planned dietary system, the protein intake had to be limited to the quantity strictly required to satisfy the specific nitrogenous needs of body maintenance, growth, pregnancy and lactation.

In adult human beings, the need for protein is very small: the body maintenance expenditure is low, for it certainly does not exceed 3 grams of nitrogen, the equivalent of 18.75 grams of protein per diem in a person of 70 kilograms. During pregnancy, women's daily needs grow to 2.3 grams and during lactation women need 16 grams a day. The different values which have been noted for the various protein foodstuffs considered separately could be widely compensated by supplements. The association with medium or poor proteins, such as those in some cereals and legumes, of a comparatively small quantity of high quality proteins raises the whole of the former. Generally speaking, in order to facilitate supplementation and raise the protein value as much as possible, it was always advisable to introduce the utmost variety into the composition of the diet.

Terroine argued that there was no need to include proteins of animal origin in the human diet, whatever the stage of life and whatever the nature of the needs to be satisfied. In his opinion, it could be useful to include such proteins when the staple food covering energy expenditure was very poor in proteins and if these were low quality. In such a case, the addition of milk or meat would raise the protein value to the required level, but the partial substitution of one legume would also have the same effect. A significant group of nutritional experts believed that the prejudice in favour of meat and the luxurious dietary habits which

---

34 Burnet, Aykroyd, 1935, p. 346.

35 Terroine, E.F., "The Protein Component in the Human Diet," *League of Nations Quarterly Bulletin of the Health Organisation*, 1936, Vol. 5, No. 3, p. 427-492.

constantly increased the consumption of meat were to be seen as absurd physiologically as they were economically.

At all stages of life and in all social groups, even during all the transient phases of existence needing special care, such as pregnancy and lactation, the indications required for guidance in the matter of nutrition are strictly the same: first, make certain that energy expenditure is amply covered; provide for this by means of foods which are rich in carbohydrates. Then, in order to raise the protein content, if necessary, to allow for the exigencies of taste, and to turn natural resources into account, add small quantities of products of animal origin, like cheese, milk, meat, and offal, bearing in mind that, economically and physiologically speaking, milk is the preferred protein food. Finally, supply, by means of fresh fruit and raw vegetables, the necessary ballast, mineral salts and vitamins.

Carbohydrate and fat requirements

No knowledge had emerged as to the optimum proportions of carbohydrates and fats in the diet, although it was accepted that they were interchangeable within wide limits. Carbohydrates were acknowledged not only to provide energy, but also to facilitate the breakdown of protein and assist the metabolism of fat.

Standards of fat intake showed wide variation, as did the intake of populations in different parts of the world. Its high calorific content reduced the amount of food needed, and was the vehicle of fat-soluble vitamins, important for breast-fed infants. Burnet and Aykroyd (1935) proposed the following standards:[36]

Standard dietaries put forward by various authorities as being suitable for average humans:

Standard dietaries put forward by various authorities as being suitable for average men

	Protein	Fat (grams)	Carbohy-drate	Calories
Voit	118	56	500	3,055
Rubner	127	52	509	3,092
Atwater	125	125	450	3,520
Advisory Committee (British Ministry)	100	100	400	3,000
Playfair	119	51	531	3,140
Tyszka	80-100	60-80	500	3,000

36 Burnet, Aykroyd, 1935, p. 348.

For children, pregnant and lactating women, as well as for those engaged in hard manual work, abundance was considered to be essential. On the contrary, the ideal of frugality was more appropriate for middle-aged and elderly men and women leading a sedentary life.[37]

Mineral salts and vitamins

As a general principle, no diet was deemed adequate by physiologists unless it contained enough mineral elements present in human tissues, those minerals taking part in metabolic actions, which need to be replaced by nutrition. Mineral deficiencies could also produce diseases. Calcium and iron were soon identified as a causal factor for diseases such as anaemia, osteoporosis and other deficiencies, and iodine deficiency was associated to goitre and cretinism. The consequences of phosphorus, calcium, iron and iodine deficits were immediately investigated and the dietary amounts of those minerals estimated. A diet rich in cereals was considered poor in phosphorus, and the absence of vitamin D, a complementary factor for rickets. The estimated amount of phosphorus in the diet was around 1.30 grams per day for the average adult, the needs of growing children being relatively higher. Most Western dietaries contained a sufficiency of phosphorus.

Calcium was considered to be the inorganic element which contributed the most to body weight. Over 99% of organic calcium is in the bones.

> Sherman and his colleagues, having made a compilation of all *calcium balance* experiments recorded in the literature, discovered that in 97 experiments, the average daily calcium output was 0.459 gram. This, Sherman takes to be the minimum requirement. Since dietary standards should be set above the minimum, he proposes a figure 50% higher – 0.68 gram – to represent the calcium requirements of the average man. The needs of children and pregnant and lactating women are higher; 1 gram has been proposed for children, and it appears that the optimum requirements of pregnant women may be as high as 1.6 grams."[38]

Experts on the physiology of nutrition linked vitamin D with the metabolic use of calcium and they therefore argued that calcium intake was especially important when the intake of vitamin D was very small, as was the case in wintertime or in countries where the sun seldom shone.

Iron had been less investigated than the previously cited minerals. Its deficiency was associated with some types of anaemia; 15 milligrams

---

[37] Burnet, Aykroyd, 1935, p. 348-349.

[38] Burnet, Aykroyd, 1935, p. 350.

was the standard daily amount recommended. Iodine deficiency was associated with endemic goitre in mountainous areas far from the sea, 25 milligrams being the estimated amount needed by an adult man weighing 70 kilos, almost half of it contained in the thyroid gland. Public health campaigns to prevent goitre were carried out in Switzerland and some areas of the United States of America: iodine compounds were administered to schoolchildren and sodium iodine was added to table salt. It was generally admitted that the prevention of goitre was ensured by the intake of 50 milligrams per year, although in endemic areas doses of 5 to 10 milligrams per week had been administered.

Some technical reports on the physiology of nutrition

An International Vitamin Conference, attended by a wide international group of experts in the physiology of nutrition, was held in London in June 1931 under the auspices of the Permanent Commission on Biological Standardisation of the League of Nations' Health Organisation.[39] A further report was published in 1934 on the international adoption of standards and units for vitamins A, B1, C and D. The conference was chaired by E. Mellanby (League of Nations) and the group of participants was integrated by J.C. Drummond (League of Nations), H. von Euler (Stockholm), L.S. Fridericia (Copenhagen), B.C.P. Jansen (Amsterdam), P. de Mattei (Pavia), E.M. Nelson (Washington), E. Poulsson (Oslo), Randoin (Paris), Steenbock (Madison), Szent-Györgyi (Szeged), Chick (League of Nations) and Aykroyd (LoN, Geneva). Other assistants were H. Brorw (Toronto), K.H. Coward (League of Nations), H.H. Dale (League of Nations), P. Hartley (League of Nations), E.M. Hume (League of Nations), A. Jung (Basel), Ch. Lormand (Paris), Rafael Méndez (Madrid), A. Morton (Liverpool), R.A. Peters (Oxford), O. Rosenheim (League of Nations), M. Tsurumi (LoN, Japan), T.A. Webster (League of Nations) and S.S. Zilva (League of Nations).

A report published in 1937 by the Technical Commission on Nutrition of the League of Nations summarised the available knowledge regarding mineral and vitamin requirements, proteins, fats, and nutritional requirements during the first year of life; the report also touched upon the nutritive value of milk and referred to some nutrition surveys on food consumption and some methods to assess the nutritional condition of infants and adolescents; it finished with an approach to nutri-

---

39 "Second Conference on Vitamin Standardisation," *League of Nations Quarterly Bulletin of the Health Organisation*, 1934, Vol. 3, p. 428-440.

tional problems in the Far East and Chile.[40] A table on the nutritive value of foods included milk, cheese, eggs, liver, fatty fish, green vegetables, raw fruits, butter, cod-liver oil, yeast, meat, root vegetables, legumes, cereals (bread, rice, nuts), sugar, jam, honey, margarine, olive and vegetable oil.

In August 1938 the Technical Commission on Nutrition of the League of Nations met in Geneva.[41] The experts convened under the chairmanship of Sir E. Mellanby, Secretary-General of the Medical Research Council, London.[42]

A series of interdependent topics were discussed:

a) The nutritive value of different cereals according to the degree of milling.

b) The influence of climate on food requirements.

c) The extent to which diets in common use fell below the standards recommended in the *Report on the Physiological Bases of Nutrition.*

As bread played a prominent part in nutrition, particularly in rural areas, and since its composition widely varied across European regions, a special study on the composition and preparation of bread was considered indispensable. This research had been conducted formerly by E.J. McDougall, of the Imperial Bureau of Animal Nutrition at the Rowett Institute (Aberdeen) and of the Basle Institute of Physiology.

Based on the importance of geo-climatic factors, the influence of climate on food requirements was a topic to include in the discussions. Starting with an analysis of the literature, the technical commission decided to contact suitable experts for this purpose. The Nutrition Research Laboratories at Coonor (India) led by W.R. Aykroyd would liaise with Far-Eastern countries and the Technical Commission. The

40 "Report by the Technical Commission on Nutrition on the Work of its third session, held in London from November 15th to 20th, 1937," *Bulletin of the Health Organisation*, 1938, Vol. 7, p. 460-502.

41 "Technical Commission on Nutrition. Report by a Special Committee which met in Geneva from August 22nd to 24th, 1938," *Bulletin of the Health Organisation*, 1938, Vol. 7, p. 667-678.

42 The participants were: W.R. Aykroyd, Director of the Nutrition Research Laboratories, Conoor, India; E.J. Bigwood, Professor of Physiology, University of Brussels; L.E. Booher, Chief Food and Nutrition Division Bureau of Home Economics, US Department of Agriculture, Washington; H. Chick, Head of the Division of Nutrition, Lister Institute, League of Nations; L.S. Fridericia, Professor of Hygiene at the University of Copenhagen; A. Mayer, Professor at the *Collège de France*, Paris; J. B. Orr, Director of the Rowett Institute of Animal Nutrition, Aberdeen; participating also as observer: W.Ph. Kennedy, Professor of Physiology at the Royal College of Medicine, Baghdad.

Committee also requested an advisory opinion concerning the feeding of refugees in countries where whole population groups were threatened with acute malnutrition, or with actual famine. Considering all these important topics, a summary of the meeting's agenda could be drafted as follows. Food requirements for infants and small incomes represented a particular point of concern. When considering special dietary needs for different social classes and age groups, expectant and nursing mothers occupied a central place for

> although it is true that our knowledge of feeding in pregnancy and lactation is elementary, it can be said with some assurance that, in regard to the health of both mother and offspring, an increase in the protective foodstuffs would have a large effect in eliminating many of the ills of pregnancy.[43]

The pre-natal period was most important from a nutritional perspective. Diet supervision in pregnant women and infants was soon included in maternity hospitals and children health care dispensaries. Nutritional experts tried to regulate the optimum diet for a pregnant woman, particular attention being paid to vitamin D, calcium and iron so as to prevent rickets and anaemia. Calcium needs in pregnant women at the last stages of pregnancy and during lactation were set as high as 1.6 grams per day.[44]

Most paediatricians agreed that breastfeeding was the best option for nourishing an infant, but its health, diet and development had to be supervised because "the causes of infant mortality… made it clear that the pernicious combination of poverty and ignorance was largely responsible for the malnutrition of infancy, as, indeed, for that seen in other stages of human life."[45] Gastrointestinal disturbances and other diseases in mothers during lactation could induce vitamin deficiency, affecting the child's health. Concerning early childhood, and pre-school and nursery age: "there is a great need to maintain the resistance of children at the highest possible level against the ravages of the infectious diseases to which they will be exposed…"[46] For the poorer social groups, who could not easily afford fresh cow's milk or dried milk preparations, breastfeeding had many advantages and minimised the risk of infection, but attention had to be paid to the fact that the quality of the mother's milk depended on the quality of her diet to a certain extent.

In the 1930s *artificial* feeding and the so-called *humanised* dried milks had improved and were well accepted both by physicians and

43 *The Problem of Nutrition*, 1936, p. 39.

44 Burnet, Aykroyd, 1935, p. 401.

45 *The Problem of Nutrition*, 1936, p. 43.

46 *The Problem of Nutrition*, 1936, p. 44.

mothers as a way to complement or replace breastfeeding without risks to the infant's health.[47] Some research on mortality and morbidity was conducted on a large sample of infants under care at the Infant Welfare Society of Chicago, in which 48.5% received breast milk only until month 9, 43% were partially breastfed and 8.5% were fed on cow's milk mixtures, all the groups receiving accessory food including orange juice, cod-liver oil and cereals at certain ages. These are the mortality and morbidity results for the three groups:[48]

	Breastfed	**Partially breast-fed**	**Artificially fed**
Percent total	48.5	43.0	8.5
Morbidity percent	37.4	53.8	63.6
Total mortality percent	6.7	27.2	66.7

Breastfeeding was associated with higher standards of health in this group of 20,000 children, although other factors could have also influenced figures. During the mid 1930s there was a tendency among paediatricians to recommend some complements to milk. Prevention of anaemia appearing at the end of the first year was the main argument. Fruit juice and cod-liver oil were given after the second month. Towards the end of the fourth month apple or banana pulp was introduced and at the end of the sixth month egg yolk and mashed vegetables. Nevertheless, milk and particularly breast milk, if possible, was considered the best option during the first nine months of infancy.[49]

A general agreement was reached: nutrition in childhood should be carefully balanced and adapted, in quantity and quality, to an organism whose condition is continually varying.[50] The total calorie allowance estimated for children reached high figures: 60 to 80 calories per kilo or even 100 depending on the author, while in average adults 40 calories per kilo were accepted. Qualitative requirements were 55% carbohydrates, 30% fats and 15% proteins, also including mineral salts, water and vitamins. It is by controlling the diet of the children, omitting nothing and not hesitating to specify even the slightest details that the

47 Burnet, Aykroyd, 1935, p. 401-402.

48 Burnet, Aykroyd, 1935, p. 402.

49 Burnet, Aykroyd, 1935, p. 402-403.

50 Lesné, E., Dreyfus-Sée, G., "Nutrition in childhood," *League of Nations Quarterly Bulletin of the Health Organisation*, 1936, Vol. 5, No. 3, p. 531-543.

doctor will help to strengthen natural resistance, to promote general development and to put them in a position to resist disease.[51]

As a result of the economic crash in 1929, a great deal of the population in most European countries saw their income wane. The situation affected the availability of foodstuffs.[52] The relationship between income, expenditure and adequate nutrition in poor families, whether employed or unemployed, became of interest for public health experts, social workers and politicians.[53] Some energy requirements calculations were published by experts, 2,500 calories representing the daily average requirement of an unemployed man:[54]

Energy requirements calculations in relation to work and family situation

	Family requirements			**% calorie reduction[a]**	
	Strenuous work	**Moderate work**	**Unemployed**	**Strenuous work**	**Moderate work**
Single man	4000	2800	2500	39	11
Man & Wife	6400	5200	4900	23	6
Man with two dependants[b]	8500	7300	7000	18	4
Man with three Dependants[c]	9400	8200	7900	13	3

[a] Calorie % reduction for the unemployed compared to preceding work situation
[b] Wife and 10-year-old-child
[c] Wife and two children at the age of five and nine.

The weekly diet described for a meaningful group of German workers would supply sufficient energy to meet the needs of an unemployed man, while quality was below the optimum though containing the necessary food factors, including inorganic salts and vitamins to maintain health and efficiency for an indefinite period. "For children and for pregnant and nursing mothers, a greater proportion of milk in the diet would be advisable, which could be included at the expense of meat and bread. A supplement of cod-liver oil would compensate for a possible

51 Lesné, Dreyfus-Sée, 1936, p. 542-543.

52 Rotberg, R.I., Raab, T.K., *Hunger and History. The Impact of Changing Food Production and Consumption Patterns of Society*, Cambridge, Cambridge University Press, 1985.

53 Aykroyd, W.R., "Diet in relation to small incomes," *League of Nations Quarterly Bulletin of the Health Organisation*, 1933, Vol. 1, p. 130-153.

54 Aykroyd, 1933, p. 134.

deficiency of vitamin A."[55] This critical situation implied that unemployed families in Germany would have to give up a large proportion of their allowances to buy an "adequate low-cost diet."

Probably, the most serious defect of working class diets in Great Britain and Ireland was the small intake of "protective" foods, milk and green vegetables, which supply proteins of high biological value, and certain vitamins and mineral salts. The small intake of butter and animal fats, carrots and green vegetables might involve a partial deficiency of vitamin A. The foods which bulk most largely in the diet were white bread, margarine, muscle meats, potatoes and jam.[56]

Subsequently to the new international situation and the rise of social problems related to diet, community feeding became a reality. The Spanish Civil War was an exceptionally critical domain, soon followed by the Second World War.[57] A meaningful part of the population received their meals in residential institutions, armies, hospitals, sanatoria, prisons, asylums, schools and similar institutions. Health authorities became engaged in ensuring satisfactory diets and public health officers assumed the supervision of institutional diets. An increasing section of the population claimed for food relief. Several systems for the provision of cheap meals appeared or extended previous experiences in most countries. In France the *soupes populaires*, and the *fourneaux économiques* were enlarged; in Germany, *Caritas Association* lent its kitchens to volunteers in 1932 in cities such as Cologne to provide meals for thousands of people. In Britain the provision of meals through central city kitchens, traditionally used for school-meals and nursing mothers, was extended and in some cities like Birmingham the *Citizens' Society* founded a number of canteens in occupational centres run by the unemployed.

Collective feeding was conceived as one of the great public services when based on scientific grounds supplied by national institutes of nutrition. Nevertheless, industrial and mass food production was considered by the experts as a real risk for the quality of foodstuffs and for the preservation of their physiological conditions. Food industries were held responsible for the partial or total elimination or destruction of vitamins.

---

55 C. von Tyszka, *Klinische Wochenschrift*, 1930, p. 142.

56 Aykroyd, 1933, p. 146.

57 Cura, M.I. del, Huertas, R., *Alimentación y enfermedad en tiempos de hambre. España, 1937-1947*, Consejo Superior de Investigaciones Cientificas, Madrid, 2007; Barona, J. L., Perdiguero E., "Health and the War. Changing schemes and health conditions during the Spanish Civil War," *Dynamis*, 2008, Vol. 28, p. 103-126.

CHAPTER 7

Nutritional Deficiencies and Malnutrition

According to dietetic views based on experimental physiology of nutrition during the interwar years, a diet mainly composed of bread, potatoes and margarine, and comparatively lacking in eggs, butter, milk and green vegetables was considered incompatible with optimum health at any age, the latter two foodstuffs being identified as *protective*. Such a diet was deficient in protein of high biological value, in vitamin A and other vitamins and calcium.[1] On the other hand, the falling milk consumption was considered to be a serious deprivation for children. It was seemingly important to realise that the dietary value of animal food beard bore little relation to their commercial quality and cost, both elements being affected by shortages and inflation. Consequently, various food-deficiency diseases, such as scurvy, beriberi, and hunger oedema, were apt to occur in those people who, while consuming a deficient diet, were forced to make severe physical efforts. An economy of energy consumption and health was settled established and the wide deep complexity of the problem foreseen:

> The problem deserves to be carefully studied, both from the national and the international point of view. While the measures proposed should counteract the psychological and physical effects of unemployment by providing the unemployed man with work the utility of which he realises and with the additional food which he needs, they may have still more far-reaching consequences if they prove to be capable of palliating the grave drawbacks of excessive industrialisation. The problem involves factors not only of an economic, social, political and agricultural nature, but still more of a dietetic and hygienic nature.[2]

Deficient nutrition and health impairment

A general feeling spread among the population about the economic depression affecting the whole world not only undermining the social foundations on which the life of nations lied, but involving serious dangers also for physical and mental health and for the survival of

1 *The Economic Depression*, 1932, p. 456.
2 *The Economic Depression*, 1932, p. 473.

millions of people, the progress made in medicine and hygiene during previous decades being threatened. Accordingly to the report of the League of Nations' Health Organisation for the yearly period October 1932 to September 1933, deficient nutrition affected to more than 50 millions. Enquiries into the state of nutrition of the unemployed were proceeding in various countries and, as we know, a conference was convened in Berlin in December 1932.[3] Indeed, in an investigation of the effects of the depression on public health, consideration had to be given to a wide range of aspects, in particular to the intensity of the economical crisis, its duration and extent, and to the working conditions, and the cost of living, to assess the influence of a plurality of factors on death and morbidity rates. To evaluate the real dimension of the threat, collecting evidence in official statistics was the best way of mapping the situation and planning a programme of action.

An important aspect referred to the organisation of health care in every country. Several political testimonies in different countries stated that it was neither rational, nor complete, or economical, the cost of medicines representing a very large item in the expenditure incurred by institutions providing medical care. The seriousness of the crisis and its influence on the impairment of economic and social conditions brought to the arena the idea of compulsory sicknesses insurance, a possibility that was generally regarded as the most rational method of organising the protection of the working classes against sickness and against the risk of malnutrition. In fact, the cost of hospital treatment was one of the most important items of expenditure in some states and therefore governments started to introduce a financial approach to the health care system, considering the idea of an exact budget calculation, uniform methods, and daily costs based on rationalisation. It is worth noting the impairment of the social and health situation of the European population and the growing regulatory intervention of the state as main factors leading to the establishment of national health services in many European countries and not only the pressure of socialist, working class unions and political parties.

A strong link between the experimental science of nutrition, public health, economy and politics was established in the period. Experts in physiology of nutrition and public health authorities became closely related because during the interwar crisis public health work in nutrition represented an extremely important part of public health activity. The threat of malnutrition became largely a social and economic problem,

3 "Report of the Health Organisation for the Period October 1932 to September 1933. IV. Economic Depression and Public Health," *League of Nations Quarterly Bulletin of the Health Organisation*, 1933, Vol. 2, p. 529-535.

and, as such, concerned politicians, economists, agriculturists, and social workers as closely as it concerned health professionals. Nutrition deficiencies became a new factor for what was perceived as *racial degeneration*, therefore nutrition, food and diet offered a wide path to medicalisation and to the social expansion of medical knowledge as a way to rationalise social relations. Social hygiene was based on a right diet for everyone.

Scientific and medical research showed that food consumed by the organism had an importance apart from the provision of energy. The physical state of the organism largely depended on its nutrition as bearing on immunological reactions. Since last decades of the 19th century, physiologists such as Claude Bernard insisted on the importance of nutrition as a fact of *organic synthesis*, which meant perpetual creation of what he conceived as a living organism's *internal environment.* Further researchers, such as the American physiologist Walter Cannon, conceptualised this internal balance as *homeostasis*. At the start of the 20th century it was generally believed that the dietary requirements of human beings were satisfied so long as they had enough to eat, and any illness from which men not hungry might suffer was ascribed to causes other than diet. Infectious diseases represented the main problem and microbes were held responsible. Nevertheless, some decades later, it was accepted that the adequacy of a dietary depended on a number of factors and mere quantitative sufficiency was considered compatible with a whole series of qualitative defects, any one of which might produce the most serious physical consequences. In the late 1920s, poverty, children's infectious diseases, and economic crisis paved the road for a new field of action. Nutrition and infection were the main references.

On the other hand, experimental and clinical research had proved an insufficient diet to lead to serious diseases as like rickets, beriberi, pellagra, dental caries, certain types of anaemia, and to open the gate to infectious diseases, including tuberculosis, the so so-called *white pest*. But the diet was not only a factor in the prevention and treatment of certain diseases; it was related as well with physical development and, in that respect, public health did not only aim to prevent populations against disease, but also to create a maximum level of well-being, nutrition becoming a central subject.

Under those circumstances, the hygienic control of foodstuffs became a key issue. Public health authorities were concerned with the protection of the public against dangerous contaminated foodstuffs and fraudulent practices in connection with the sale of food and the feeding of population groups in schools, factories, prisons, asylums, naval and military establishments and also in any commercial transaction.[4] In war times, governments had to feed large armies whose physique and morale had to be maintained at all costs, and at the same time responsibility for providing food for the civilian population had to be assumed, a hard challenge to be successfully faced in time of shortage.

As a consequence of the economic crisis, unemployment and poverty had imposed on governments enormous responsibilities in the sphere of public assistance, one of the most urgent being the combat against defective diseases and malnutrition. The emergency situations produced by the war, post-war and the depression had helped to make clear the importance of public health nutrition work in normal times. In many European countries concerned governments controlled the food availability and the nutritional conditions of the population. State central administrations extended their programmes of action under the influence of public measures and regulations, so that nutrition was being given more and more attention in the field of public health.[5] Governmental involvement was easy to understand in a context of emergency, but it was becoming even more systematic for public health and economic reasons. In the 1930s vast numbers of human beings were malnourished or undernourished, and, indeed, famine itself had not yet disappeared, still remaining a threat.[6] But the situation would only worse as a consequence of the war, first in Spain and then in most European regions.

Although the effects of the crisis had not yet been reflected in vital and epidemiological statistics, several indications of increased morbidity among the unemployed and their families suggested a deterioration of their state of nutrition, especially among the social groups badly hit by the crisis. The situation was growing worse, and the resources of the unemployed and assisted persons were so scanty in certain regions that they no longer sufficed to procure an adequate diet.[7]

---

4 Guillem-Llobat, Perdiguero, 2006, p. 33-40.

5 Bernabeu-Mestre, J. *et al.*, "La alimentación como problema sanitario: nutrición y salud pública en la España de la primera mitad del siglo XX," in *VIII Congreso de la ADEH*, Maó, 2007, 63 p.; Bernabeu-Mestre, J., Galiana, M.E., Esplugues, J.X. and Cid, P., "Overexploitation, malnutrition and stigma in a women's illness: chlorosis in contemporary Spanish medicine (1877-1936)," in Harris, B., Gálvez, L., Machado, E. (eds.), *Gender and wellbeing in Europe: historical and contemporary perspectives*, Ashgate, Hampshire, 2009, p. 154-171.

6 Burnet, Aykroyd, 1935, p. 323-474.

7 "The most Suitable Methods of Detecting Malnutrition Due to the Economic Depression, The Conference held at Berlin from December 5th to 7th, 1932," *League of Nations Quarterly Bulletin of the Health Organisation*, 1933, Vol. 1, p. 116-129.

Medical patterns to define malnutrition

The Health Committee of the League of Nations decided to establish contact between the experts responsible for the enquiries at the time, proceeding to reach an agreement on how the state of nutrition could be determined by means of a clinical examination of a standard type to be decided upon. A Conference convened for this purpose in Berlin in December 1932, chaired by Professor E. Gorter, the director of the Children's Clinic of Leyden University (Netherlands).[8]

Two possible ways of action were discussed at the Conference. One was to study the nature and quantity of foodstuffs consumed by the individuals under examination, discussing records of diet and consumption, and making a decision about whether their diet was adequate or not. The second option was based on clinical examination with a view to determining physical condition by direct exploration. Under such critical circumstances, the second method was regarded as the most reliable to obtain a picture of the situation. These medical examinations had obviously to be applied to a sufficiently large number of people from the various classes of the unemployed and needy groups, comparing data with groups of persons belonging to the same class, whose incomes and living conditions had been unaffected by the crisis.[9]

If the number of unemployed individuals was considerable, other tests, i.e. anaemia, fatigability, pulse rate, signs of avitaminosis (xerophtalmia, rickets, oedema, etc.), could also be conducted to a lesser extent. For the organisation of the enquiries, the agencies conducting them were official public health and social hygiene services comprised of doctors, visiting nurses, and social workers with the necessary expertise and personal skills to ensure the best results.

Impelled by the need to determine nutritional deficiencies according to scientific patterns, in 1936 a general programme of research into biological measurements and tests for the definition of states of malnutrition was published by H. Laugier.[10] In spite of the hard methodological difficulties, some interesting points were emphasised in this report in

---

8 The Conference was attended by representatives from Austria (E. Nobel), Belgium (D.L.J. Gilbert), United Kingdom (Janet M. Campbell and A.F. Hurst), Denmark (Th. Madsen), France (J. Parisot), Germany (C. Hamel, E. Atzler, G. von Bergmann, W. Bansi, O. Martineck, P. Stefani and H. Zondeck), Italy (C. Gini) and USA (K.D. Blackfan and J.R. Murlin) and several members of the German Reichstag.

9 "The most Suitable Methods," 1933, p. 119.

10 Laugier, H., "General Programme of Research into Biological Measurements and Tests for the Definition of States of Malnutrition," *League of Nations Quarterly Bulletin of the Health Organisation*, 1936, Vol. 5, No. 3, p. 505-530.

order to make the practical screening of malnutrition possible. If accurate information was available concerning the weight of the person examined before the period of malnutrition, the ratio between the weight at the moment of checking and the previous weight constituted the basic criterion. In the absence of such data, some alternative measures could orient the diagnosis, such as Bouchard's index for adults and Pirquet's index for children. The amount of subcutaneous adipose tissue was also to be ascertained, but always taking into account that some obese individuals do not loose weight even if they eat very little and, conversely, there are thin people who do not put on weight notwithstanding a copious food intake.

Research in connection with the physiological effects of fasting might have shown regularities determined by urine analysis, a very valuable means to establish malnutrition indices. Unfortunately, there was a lack of such investigations and, besides, they had never been applied to determine the state of malnutrition. Some clinical signs could point to deficient nutrition, such as the loss of muscular energy and the capacity for sustained effort – reduced in a state of malnutrition –, but they were mainly studied in connection with unusual movements.

All the experimental evidence seemed to prove that an undernourished person reacted to re-nourishment rapidly and positively. The weight increases, and so does the basal metabolism, the pulse quickens and the blood pressure rises as motor capacities improve. Moreover, a series of additional tests could be made on a comparative basis before and after this feeding up period. A test consisted of meals rich in proteins. It had been noticed that undernourished persons retained nitrogen, as this element was not found in their urine in sufficient quantities. A glycosemia rate was also considered to be helpful. The general aim was to translate into laboratory indices the biological negative effects of a deficient diet.

The biological supervision of food, especially of its vitamin content, was to become one of the experimental possibilities to modify and improve nutritional qualities through an artificial vitaminisation of foodstuffs.[11] The first technical challenge to solve was the preservation of vitamins, because industrial processes were not free of risks. Some evidence showed that the permanent and excessive ingestion of artificially vitaminised foods had drawbacks over time, and accidents were reported in France, Italy and England. Randoin argued for the strict

11 Randoin, L., "On the necessity for a biological supervision of food (with Special Reference to its Vitamin Content)," *League of Nations Quarterly Bulletin of the Health Organisation, V (3)*, (1936), p. 493-504.

suppression of advertisements exaggerating the positive effects of vitamins, for the expression of vitamin contents in food in international units, and for the establishment of effective control on artificial vitaminisation by means of international regulations. Rather than an advantage, some industrial techniques affecting food had become a risk.

Surveys showed that during the 1930s the problem of nutrition varied widely from one part of the world to another. In some countries, an adequate diet was still probably within the reach of the majority of the population while in others practically all lived but little above bare subsistence level. In some countries, food prices were relatively low, but in others they were high in relation to incomes. National surveys were recommended, since local differences implied that nutrition policies must vary in different areas, their goal being to ensure that all sections of the population had an adequate diet: sufficient of energy-bearing and protective foods for optimum health.[12]

Experts reported that food habits were gradually changing in the right direction, and "those communities, on the whole, are now consuming, in addition to the indispensable foods of high energy value, more milk and dairy products, more fruit and more vegetables than a generation ago."[13] Improvement was said to derive from understanding of dietary needs, but the movement to better nutrition had not gone far enough. Once again, popular culture and tradition were faced to scientific knowledge and, according to the nutritionists' point of view, poverty and ignorance were considered to be main obstacles to progress, and disparity of prices and incomes a factor increasing difficulties. Indeed, nutrition policy was required to achieve two goals: the consumption of those products recommended as essential by experimental science, but also an improved supply, which required agriculture and commerce to adapt to new demands and cultural patterns derived from scientific knowledge.

Admitting that nutrition was a national problem in most countries was the point of departure for any solution. An extra effort had to be made to convince the public opinion. More than ever, politicians became aware of the necessity for bringing together scientists, public health experts, economists, agricultural experts, consumers' representatives, teachers and administrators in some kind of national nutrition committees recognising the importance of integrating agricultural, educational, health and economical policies.[14] European governments

---

12 *Final report*, 1937, p. 32.

13 *Final report*, 1937, p. 32.

14 *Final report*, 1937, p. 36-38.

afforded direct relief especially to the unemployed, and the extension of such social interventions was considered extremely important in order to improve the population's health status bearing in mind that the problem of malnutrition was urgent. Many governments adopted measures of direct assistance to supplement the diets of the more exposed, especially to prevent malnutrition in childhood by means of giving milk to infants, children, adolescents and expectant and nursing mothers.

From the perspective of social assistance, school meals were to play an important role in a context of dietary policies based on public and private provision of food needs. The crisis forced modern states to become directly committed to intervention on private habits, but also on public and private institutions: school canteens, hospital meals, charitable and benevolent institutions, relief centres, army, navy, prisons and other state services and institutions. Public and private authorities assumed responsibilities for the provision of meals, trying to ensure that all nutrient constituents as defined by experimental science were provided.

Medical science and hygiene had made progress since the second half of the 19th century concerning the infective nature of many diseases. But people's physical condition was still considered to be far below the accepted standard.

> [...] and the more recent advances in medical science have established the fact that this inferiority is largely due to imperfect nutrition [...] At the same time, the discoveries of the first three decades of the twentieth century leading to the *newer knowledge of nutrition* had shown with ever increasing certainty that inadequate nutrition played an excessive proportion of under-developed school-children and adolescents and the poor health and small output of a large number of workers. Deficiencies in diet and diseases of nutritional origin could be observed, not only among urban populations, but also among dwellers in country districts, and not only in poor or primitive countries, but also in the rich nations with an old and highly developed civilisation.[15]

In all Western countries, the average diet of the population had become increasingly diversified from the beginning of the 20th century. There had been a tendency for the consumption of dairy products, eggs, fruits and vegetables to increase; and the great staples, such as cereals and potatoes, had come to constitute a smaller proportion of human foodstuffs. The fact that a larger amount of the total calorie requirements were derived from the highly protective foods represented a great nutritional advance and showed that there was a natural tendency on the part

---

[15] *Final report*, 1937, p. 59-60.

of consumers to become more aware of the importance of rational nutrition as far as economic circumstances so permitted. An exception usually mentioned was the increasing consumption of sugar in certain countries.

The most notable trends, apart from the remarkable increase in sugar consumption, were the continuous rise of milk, butter and eggs, the steady fall in bread consumption and the post-war decline in the consumption of potatoes. It seemed clear, from the examples given, that the average diet of the urban working classes in Western countries tended to include larger amounts of protective foods. Instead of the general improvements and changes in feeding habits, the diet of a substantial portion of the population remained deficient in essential nutritive elements, giving way to an unquestionable problem of malnutrition even in countries with the highest standards of living.

The changing content of the diet of Western countries was not an accident; it corresponded to a genuine change both in physiological requirements and in the possibility to satisfy them. Most of the experts believed that the principal factors were the reduction in the expenditure of muscular energy caused by unemployment, increased mechanisation in industry and agriculture, and the reduction in the hours of work on the one hand and the rising number of those engaged in commerce, trade, clerical work, administration and other quasi-sedentary occupations, on the other. By far, labourers doing heavy manual work obviously spent more energy than do machine – tenders or office – workers. An ever smaller fraction of the population was engaged in the primary industries such as agriculture and forestry, and a constantly increasing proportion in manufacturing, trade, transportation, clerical and professional occupations.

Other factors were also involved. Among them, the experts' commissions mentioned the improvement in housing conditions, which reduced the amount of food required for keeping the body at a constant temperature, and the increased use of automobiles and mechanic transport, which reduced the amount of walking, and less energy was being spent as a result. According to nutritional expertise, the growing vogue of outdoor sports and physical exercise meant, on the contrary, an increase in muscular effort and exposure to cold. As a consequence, changes in the character nature of work, leisure activities and the way of life in modern civilisation and urban living resulted in changes in food requirements.

Economic facts were also to be taken into consideration: the foodstuffs which have tended to feature in the diet were usually more expensive than those they had displaced, and the so-called modern diet became dearer than the diet of previous decades, which had uneven effects upon everyday life in times of crisis.

The influence of poverty and the social consequences of the economic depression in some aspects like unemployment resulted in an impaired diet. Since the quality of the diet was closely related to its cost, the economic crisis represented a threat leading to nutritional problems and starvation. Even though animal foods were still widely available in some countries, the general tendency towards an inexpensive diet caused people to overlook nutrition. On the other hand, as we have seen, experts in public health associated poverty to ignorance of how available resources could be combined to the best advantage.

The effects of malnutrition caused by poverty and exclusion took some time to reach a clinical level, becoming apparent after a long interval. "A child whose diet contains too high a proportion of cheap carbohydrates may retain a *normal* weight for a fairly long time, even though a state of anaemia and debility has already set in. The actual duration of the inadequate nutrition is a very important factor."[16] However, it was widely recognised that even among the very poor the diet could be influenced by factors other than income, such as maternal efficiency and cultural habits. Relief was necessary as a social tool, but also education in marketing, values, cooking and methods of preservation. Housewife efficiency was considered to be a keystone of the problem of nutrition during the economic crisis and it mostly depended upon educating mothers. All instruments had to be put in action to reach this target: campaigns, films, lectures, radio. Mothers became a key player in the process of civilisation, and changing dietary habits was a part of it.

In the two Conferences of Experts convened in 1932 to discuss nutrition problems, a great deal of attention was paid to poverty and malnutrition, as the crisis had widely spread. The first conference on dietary standards took place in Rome[17] and the second one, held in Berlin, discussed physical standards and clinical and physiological methods to detect malnutrition. Since nutrition had become a basic part of public health, governments adopted measures of protection and assistance with regard to food supplies. In some countries, specific legislation to guarantee food supply to the population was applied.[18] The prosperity of

---

16 Burnet, Aykroyd, 1935, p. 384.

17 "Conference of Experts for the Standardisation of Certain Methods used in making Dietary Studies. Held in Rome on September 2nd and 3rd, 1932," *League of Nations Quarterly Bulletin of the Health Organisation*, 1932, Vol. 1, No. 1, p. 477-483.

18 "Report on the Physiological Bases," 1936, p. 66.

farmers, peasants and agricultural workers was considered to be an essential element in any policy intended to improve nutrition, and agricultural technologies and practices had to be adapted to meet the new requirements.

The adaptation to the new situation required to satisfy new demands on the basis of protective foods rather than energy producing ones. The experts of the League of Nations' Health Committee believed that the trend of dietary habits in Western countries would coincide with an evolution of agricultural production, which would benefit rural populations and might also contribute to a resumption of steady economic relations between the nations.[19]

The meeting held in Rome in September 1932, was presided by E.P. Cathcart, Professor of Physiology at the University of Glasgow, expert on quantitative methods of nutrition. Participants included a selected international group of physiologists, clinicians and statisticians interested in all aspects of dietetics. They discussed some problems in connection with the study of human nutrition with the aim of achieving more general uniformity in research techniques used in family dietary enquiries. In their attempt to lay down family scales, the participants believed that the food intake of a manual worker was to be usually greater than that of his wife and children, or that of a sedentary worker. They proposed the use of two different scales: one for families in which the man was engaged in heavy work activity and another one for families in which he was less strenuously employed. It was thought desirable for any scale of family coefficients to accurately express the intake of the different family members according to sex and age. But the important point was to secure general agreement on a particular scale, even if that scale was not strictly accurate. Agreement on scales would allow comparisons between countries, regions and social groups.

The problem of comparing results made the group of experts aware of methodological discussion. The technique of dietary studies was to be discussed considering the optimum duration of enquiries, the relative advantages of direct and indirect enquiries, the methods to be adopted in dealing with household waste, and physiological needs.[20] A few years later, Bigwood guidelines were accepted as a model to follow.

An international food policy, as claimed for by the international committees, also required the international unification of the technical

19 "Report on the Physiological Bases," 1936, p. 95.

20 "Current Notes on the Work of the Health Organisation. Conference on Nutrition," *League of Nations Quarterly Bulletin of the Health Organisation*, 1932, Vol. 1, No. 1, p. 311.

analysis and control of food quality of foodstuffs, setting up standards of reference and specifications for grading foods of all kinds according to quality. Bearing in mind that each country had previously developed its own regulations, and institutions for the control and expertise, a coordination of the nutrition work done by different authorities was recommended.[21] Based on the collection of records about consumption by families of different occupational groups with different income levels, international comparative records were to become essential in verifying to what extent national dietaries fell short of the new standards. Scientific standards aimed to become references of authority in the process of disciplining the economy and dietary habits. The Mixed Committee of the three international organisations argued that national statistics on food supply and consumption should be improved and that the International Institute of Agriculture should collect information regarding supply, national consumption and prices.[22]

We shall comment in a later chapter that the Mixed Committee also offered a survey on the post-war nutritional situation in Europe, South Africa, Australia, Siam and Turkey, including recommendations and measures to improve nutrition in particular sections of the population, such as mothers and infants, school-age children and young people, adults, unemployed, and army and navy dietaries. They also suggested measures to reduce prices and make available to consumers foodstuffs at reduced prices, and measures for ensuring the quality of foodstuffs, experimental and clinical research on nutrition, education and popular instruction to prompt a change in dietary practices. The International Institute of Agriculture in Rome provided information on foodstuffs consumption, particularly of milk and fresh vegetables in large cities, as well as on trends in production and the evolution of prices. The international programme also collected records on financial aspects of assistance to national agriculture in various countries and studied wholesale and retail prices, particularly of protective foods, relating prices to trends in production and consumption in different countries. These technical reports aided to shape an international landscape, put forward comparison criteria and to discuss the way to homogenize patterns of intervention.[23]

During the Depression, it was thought that general incomes would rise sooner or later and therefore special actions had to be taken to

---

21 Guillem-Llobat, X., *El control de la qualitat dels aliments. El cas valencià en el context internacional (1878-1936)*, Valencia, PUV, 2007.

22 "Report on the physiological bases," 1936, p. 97-98.

23 *Nutrition in various countries*, Series of League of Nations Publications, Geneva, 1936 [Technical Report A.12(b).1936.II.B], p. 269.

improve the nutrition of particular groups of the community. Adjustment and adaptation appeared as keystones. The demand for protective foods was likely to grow more than the demand for those chiefly consumed for their high energy value. In attempting to define the effort of adaptation required of agriculture, particular attention was drawn to two points: nutrition policy should not involve a rapid transformation in the existing structure of national agricultural systems and, as nutrition policy moved towards its objective of an adequate diet for all, an increase in the demand for all classes of agricultural products would be expected. The prosperity of farmers, peasants and agricultural workers was therefore considered an essential starting point within policies directed towards improved nutrition, and agricultural practice should be adapted to meet the new requirements of better nutrition.[24]

The Technical Commission on Nutrition of the League of Nations Health Organisation held in its third session in November 1937.[25] In the first two sessions, the Commission had endeavoured to define, "in the light of modern conceptions of physiology," what principles of nutrition would most suitably ensure the rational development and optimum maintenance of the human organism. The result of its work was the *General Report on the Physiological Bases of Nutrition*, published in September 1938. We have already discussed its contents in some detail in a previous chapter. At the end of the report ten important topics were listed for further study, most of them regarding the nutrition of children and standards: 1. Assessment of the nutritional state of children in different countries and regions; 2. Nutritive food requirements during the first year of life; 3. Minimum vitamin and mineral requirements; 4. Minimum fat requirements; 5. Nutritive and supplementary values of protein-containing foods, to determine to what extent animal proteins are necessary for growth and health; 6. Relative nutritive value of cereals according to the degree of milling; 7. To what extent increasing consumption of sugar is detrimental to health; 8. Influence of climate on food requirements; 9. To what extent common diets fall below the standards recommended in the report, and 10. Definition of the optimum amount of milk consumed at different ages.

The commission's report was strongly influential. It was made public and communicated to the learned societies and scientific institutions of several countries with a view to securing their observations and co-operation in the aforesaid studies. Nevertheless, from a practical per-

---

24 *The Problem of Nutrition*, 1936, p. 84.

25 "Report on the work of the Health Organisation between June 1937 and May 1938, and on its 1938 Programme. 4. Nutrition," *League of Nations Bulletin of the Health Organisation*, 1938, Vol. 7, p. 642-647.

spective the Commission could not cover all ten questions in a biennium and so concentrated on the first five.

At the same period, a meeting on the *Nutritional state of children* was held in December 1936. In their final report the experts recommended to assess the state of nutrition of large numbers of children, and to further develop somatometric, clinical and physiological tests, designed to detect the first signs of malnutrition at the earliest possible moment. Nutritive food requirements during the first year of life were also discussed. Attention was paid to this subject in a previous chapter.

The following meetings of the technical commission were devoted to discussing physiological concepts such as minimum vitamin, mineral and fat requirements, and nutritive and supplementary values of protein-containing foods, and determining to what extent animal proteins were necessary for growth and health. When the commission met in November 1937, a careful review was made of existing knowledge on such questions, and the resulting findings were incorporated in the first four chapters of a new report. It came to the conclusion that it was essential to carry out a study of mineral metabolism including the factors influencing the utilisation of calcium and phosphorus, the proportion of assimilable iron in the various foodstuffs, the quantities of iron necessary for adults of both sexes, especially for women during pregnancy and lactation, and the assimilation of iron by children. Fears of anaemia and nutritional deficiencies were always present in the agenda.

In the last meeting held in November 1937, the technical commission on nutrition endeavoured to show, in the light of recent research, why milk was a foodstuff of such paramount importance, especially during growth in childhood, and emphasised the need to eliminate the dangers of milk as a vehicle for bacterial infection. Considering that the last five points were still being surveyed "a study of the food intake of urban and rural populations will therefore play a prominent part in the programme of work for 1938."[26]

Between June 1938 and April 1939 the work of the Health Organisation Technical Commission on Nutrition was directed along two main lines. It changed the geographical perspective, previously focused on Western countries and, in pursuance of a recommendation adopted by the General Advisory Health Council in 1937, it was to undertake the study of nutrition in Asia and tropical countries generally. In addition, the Commission was to deal with qualitative and quantitative surveys designed to bring any nutritional deficiencies to light. Moreover, the

---

26 "Report on the work of the Health Organisation," 1938, p. 646.

Commission also followed the logical outcome of the previous activities.[27]

With particular regard to the Far East and to tropical countries, the Committee considered that fuller information was required on dietary habits, the incidence of diseases connected with dietary deficiencies, and the nutritional value of local foods.[28] As a starting point, it reached some general conclusions on national programmes and urged certain adjustments in the sphere of agriculture to increase the production of protective foods. However, more complete dietary surveys were to be made to find food supplies in the rural and urban areas of several countries using statistics on production and consumption as a main tool.

Three types of enquiries into the state of nutrition of populations were suggested:

1. Large-scale demographic investigations, a record being made of age and sex, physical appearance, height, and weight of each subject. That is to say, a sort of individual chart containing general anthropometric features.

2. A second level including more detailed investigations covering a limited number of individuals. Core features of children's diet, exhaustive medical examination of individuals, economic and social position of the family, somatometric data, photographs, and tests to detect pre-deficiency conditions among other data were suggested.

3. Third level consisting of bio-topological investigations regarding morphological characteristics and biological functions, as well as psychological examination.

During its August session, the attention of the Special Committee was drawn to the fact that, even in Europe, disturbing conditions existed in which the problem was no longer to lay down the bases for a satisfactory diet, but rather to prevent the population from dying from starvation. This was, more particularly, the position of Spain in 1938, affected by two years of war. To cope with it, the Society of Friends sought guidance in the preparation of an emergency diet for the refugees. The Committee suggested a diet of this character mainly composed of whole wheat, brewer's dried yeast, cod-liver oil and various salts. This emergency diet was so designed as to include vitamins and essential inorganic constituents. At the same time, the Committee pointed out that such a diet was at most adequate to sustain life and to prevent the ap-

---

27 "Report on the work of the Health Organisation between June 1938 and April 1939 and on its 1939 programme. B. Nutrition," *League of Nations Bulletin of the Health Organisation*, 1939, Vol. 8, p. 27-32.

28 "Report on the work of the Health Organisation," 1939, p. 29.

pearance, during a limited period, of the more serious effects of malnutrition. Nevertheless it should not be interpreted as a permanent dietary pattern. It could only be looked upon as an emergency diet, to be supplemented at the earliest possible moment by fresh foods.[29]

[29] "Report on the work of the Health Organisation," 1939, p. 32.

CHAPTER 8

Rural Dietaries in Europe

E.J. McDougall's report on rural Europe

A specific report on food habits in rural populations in Europe was prepared by the experts' commission on nutrition of the League of Nations' Health Organisation. Rural health, dietaries and living conditions became a main point of interest in time of crisis. According to all surveys, rural communities and dietaries were extremely different in the varied rural areas of Europe. Yet they showed certain common characteristics as contrasted with urban dietaries and living conditions.[1] Although, in each geographical area of Europe there existed particular records in peasants' food habits, surveys in different rural areas evidenced certain similarities. The chief characteristic of rural diets underlined in the surveys was monotony, since the average peasant household only used a limited number of foodstuffs. From a nutritional point of view, this was clearly a disadvantage, since, in a more varied diet, there was less risk of being deprived of one or more essential foods, particularly minerals and vitamins. In rural communities seasonal variations were considerable, but day-to-day dietaries often lacked variety for most of the year.

The improvement in communications and means of transport was indeed an advantage for food trade and commercial distribution, but it might at the same time imply a nutritional disadvantage for primitive isolated rural areas in as much as they allowed selling their products to towns. This meant that certain foodstuffs traditionally consumed were being kept for sale and not consumed at home any more. McDougall's report attributed to this reason, the fact that the level of consumption of animal foodstuffs was reported to be higher in certain poor parts of Europe than in more developed neighbouring areas. It was not ignorance but economic necessity which prevented peasants from eating the meat, eggs and the dairy products they produced. In most districts these foodstuffs were considered luxuries and only prosperity introduced them into

1 [McDougall, E.J.] "Rural dietaries in Europe," *League of Nations Quarterly Bulletin of the Health Organisation*, 1939, Vol. 8, No. 3, p. 470-497. [C.H./Com.Exp.Alim./59, 25 p.].

peasantry dietaries.[2] Nevertheless, local traditions played a meaningful role and often this important factor was not taken into consideration in most of the expert reports. Goat or sheep-milk cheese was eaten in poor rural areas whereas in more developed ones cheese production was usually sold in towns.

> Thus, apart from certain isolated areas where meat, fish or milk products are the most abundant foodstuffs, and where the lack of transport facilities prevents a profitable sale of these products, the great majority of rural people sell most of the animal foodstuffs which they produce, and live on a diet largely composed of cereals and vegetables.[3]

Again, education was pointed out as the key element to improving rural nutrition. Quite often, when talking about dietaries and food consumption, popular culture and scientific knowledge confronted one other. McDougall's report on rural dietaries stated that: "The majority of rural housewives in Europe know little or nothing of the principles of nutrition, and they might frequently be able to feed their families more adequately if they knew the relative value of different foodstuffs."[4] Nevertheless, cultural habits attaching to the consumption of certain foods varied considerably between countries and regions depending on availability, religious beliefs and local traditions. During the interwar period many Western countries started campaigns to instruct the rural housewife, who was considered to be the keystone to changes in traditional habits contrary to new scientific ideas.[5]

Apart from education as a tool to change habits, state relief in the form of food supplies was often given to destitute rural families in many European countries after the 1929 crisis. School meals and public canteens for unemployed and poor people spread in many rural areas in Europe. However, two levels of action were on the arena to orient political strategies. The first level was linked to the urgent necessity to overcome shortages, wrong dietary habits and nutrition deficiencies. But this was not enough, because the economic dimension of severe deficiencies in rural nutrition could only be tackled by agricultural and economic readjustments, both nationally and internationally.

> The first requirement of the average European peasant is to produce, with the greatest economy of land and of labour, foodstuffs which will supply the maximum energy value which he needs for hard physical work. For this reason, cereals, which are the cheapest form of energy-providing foodstuffs to

---

2 [McDougall, E.J.] "Rural dietaries," 1939, p. 475.

3 [McDougall, E.J.] "Rural dietaries," 1939, p. 472.

4 [McDougall, E.J.] "Rural dietaries," 1939, p. 475.

5 [McDougall, E.J.] "Rural dietaries," 1939, p. 474-475.

> produce, for the basis of most peasants dietaries. The type of cereal used varies from wheat in Western Europe and the Danube Basin, to rye in Northern Europe, and maize and barley in parts of Eastern and South-eastern Europe; but whether the cereal grown (or bought) is wheat, rye, barley, oats or maize, it is used in the great majority of peasants households throughout Europe as the basis of every meal.[6]

Certain exceptions were reported for mountain regions of the Balkans, Sub-Carpathian Russia and Scandinavia, where cereals could not be easily grown and the diet was made up of whichever variety of vegetables could be produced (potatoes, beans, etc.) and animal foodstuffs available. Since these foods were usually more expensive than cereals, those populations were frequently underfed, unless some complementary income was found or state relief provided through special means such as wagon-loads of cereals.

According to McDougall's report, the preponderance of cereals in the rural dietary was most marked in Central, Eastern and South-Eastern Europe, where the cereal provision of energy was estimated to be 80% to 90% of the total diet.[7] His report concluded that the high proportion of cereals intake decreased as the peasant population became more prosperous and had been substantially reduced in Western and Northern Europe for a series of agricultural and climatic causes. On the other hand, in those European regions identified by nutritionists as "the more primitive areas," cereals were not only eaten as bread but also simply ground to a rough meal and cooked with water as groats, porridge, polenta or cakes.[8]

The second most important foodstuffs in rural areas of Europe were some vegetables of a high energy-providing value. In rural Ireland, Poland or Germany, potatoes were even more important in the diet than cereals, while in the Balkan Region and Central Europe, beans constituted a regular source of calories in the rural dietary, according to data in McDougall's report.

Less homogeneous seemed to be the amount and varieties of meat eaten from one region to another. The consumption of meat was said to depend on the prosperity of the peasantry and on cultural habits, but the importance of certain animals for human survival in many rural districts is well-known. Some of them delivered milk, wool and other stuffs fundamental for rural families. In other cases, animal products took part of rural economy, as well as rural dietaries. The case of Spanish peas-

---

6 [McDougall, E.J.] "Rural dietaries," 1939, p. 470-471.

7 [McDougall, E.J.] "Rural dietaries," 1939, p. 470.

8 [McDougall, E.J.] "Rural dietaries," 1939, p. 471.

antry and farmers in relation to pork consumption is paradigmatic. The so so-called *matanza* [slaughter of the pig] constituted a big feast, an essential event in many rural districts, associated to old traditions and probably religious beliefs. One should conclude that the insistence of nutritionists on the lack of meat consumption among poor social groups in rural districts is not always acceptable; sausages, most animal viscera and organs, blood, intestines, all took part of popular rural dietaries in different ways and proportions. Animal products were not always a luxury for many peasants in Southern Europe; medical topographies and official reports confirm this fact.

However, McDougall insisted on the idea that poorer farmers in the poorest parts of Europe would only eat meat on feast days, just a few times a year, while the more prosperous peasants in those poor regions used to eat it once or twice a week. This was probably true for meat, but not for all animal products supplying animal proteins. On the contrary, he reports that, in the most prosperous areas of Western Europe, the poorest peasants ate meat once a week, while prosperous farmers had two or three meat meals daily. Was it mainly a matter of prosperity? He stated: "The consumption of milk also varies enormously from one part of Europe to another. In Finland and Latvia, the rural population is reported to drink a litre of milk per head per day, while in Hungary, Romania and Yugoslavia there are districts where peasant families drink practically no milk at all."[9]

Indeed, not only McDougall's report but also other nutritionists insisted on the idea that production and consumption were sometimes dissociated. The case of milk was frequently mentioned because it was reported that peasants who produced milk, butter and cheese, regarded these products primarily as market goods and not as essential foodstuffs for their own families. McDougall cited the striking example of Danish farmers producing butter for export and buying margarine for their own consumption. In many rural areas, milk was considered an essential foodstuff for newborns and infants, but was absolutely out of an adult's diet. Due to the insistence of rural doctors and hygienists on the benefits of milk consumption, it has been reported in Spanish rural districts a widely extended popular belief was reported that associated milk to a medical product, a sort of medicine for sick people, rather than a foodstuff.

Surveys and reports by hygienists and nutritional experts showing evident deficiencies in rural dietaries put some questions to historical evaluation. Cultural habits were seldom positively considered as a

---

9 [McDougall, E.J.] "Rural dietaries," 1939, p. 472.

fundamental element of rural dietaries. Everything contrary to the new scientific discourse was labelled by scientists as *ignorance.* To what an extent were experts legitimated to talk about ignorance as a main cause of nutritional deficiency, especially when cultural habits were the principal tool for survival in traditional societies? Was it really a lack of scientific knowledge or was it cultural habits and economic necessity that prevented peasants from having meat, eggs and the dairy products they produced? In most cases, certain products were not included in traditional rural dietaries and it seems reasonable to wonder if such foodstuffs were considered to be a luxury or simply they were not part of family traditional cuisine. Was prosperity really the path to introduce new foodstuffs into the peasantry dietary? Undoubtedly, cultural habits also played a role to a great extent. But habits were often put down to *ignorance* by the experts. McDougall remarks that such valuable foodstuffs as whey and blood were wasted in certain areas while consumed in others. It is remarkable how new scientists identified science as knowledge and considered culture and popular habits on the side of ignorance, showing the authoritarian mentality of the positivistic approach trying to civilise the ignorant.

Other factors were also considered in nutritional surveys in relation to the urban-rural divide. Rural dietaries tended to be affected by much greater seasonal dependence than in urban areas, because most peasant families relied on what was grown locally and urban areas received stuffs from different places. In those cases, the diet used to be at its best in late summer and autumn, a period in which a wide variety of fruits was available and cereals, vegetables, eggs and milk products were more abundant. During this period, the diet of peasants was almost an ideal diet, particularly in areas where milk was abundantly drunk. Fruits and vegetables were eaten in adequate amounts; milk and meat products were easily available. Just the opposite was true in spring in Central and Eastern rural Europe; it was during this season that most health problems associated to the diet appeared, such as pellagra, scurvy, night blindness, rickets and others. During the hard periods of the year, rural diets tended to be deficient in fruits, fresh green vegetables and animal foodstuffs. In addition, religious fasting further impoverished the winter diet, as no animal products were eaten and the global intake of proteins decreased.[10] Accordingly to the expert's approach, to increase the consumption of fresh fruits and vegetables, it was necessary to learn how to preserve them for winter use, avoiding much of the crop being wasted. The conservation of fresh foodstuffs became an important challenge for many rural areas.

---

[10] [McDougall, E.J.] "Rural dietaries," 1939, p. 470 *passim*.

McDougall's report coincided with other experts in the idea that the only special advantage of rural dietaries over urban ones was that food in the countryside was usually consumed in fresher, more natural condition, something important for cereals "which are usually eaten as highly refined white flour in the towns, while, in most parts of Europe, the rural populations still eat whole-grain cereals."[11] The difference between refined and wholemeal flour was undoubtedly considered of great nutritional significance, especially in rural regions, where bread and other forms of cereal food formed the basis of the diet. Nutritionists knew that the proportion of minerals and vitamins decreased largely in refined white flour, something that might not be important in urban varied diets, but, on the contrary, it was probably meaningful in the more restricted rural dietaries. In many cases, nutritionists shared a critical and suspicious attitude towards the quality control of industrialised food at a time when a debate was open on the use of colourings and other additives requiring further regulation.[12] Among other losses, minerals and vitamins were considered by some physiologists to be lost as a result of industrial processing. This would not be important in urban more varied diets but, once more, it could be a serious threat in the more restricted rural diets.

The problem of dietary habits

One of the main sources of confrontation between popular habits and the new expertise was the feeding of specific groups of the population, such as infants, young children, and pregnant and nursing mothers. A great amount of technical reports, surveys and experimental research were devoted to the nutrition of these particular groups of population. Although infants were usually breastfed longer in rural areas than in towns and cities, experience showed that rickets was widespread in most rural regions. This paradox was explained by hygienists as a consequence of deficiencies in the mother's diet, which was too poor to provide the child with the necessary minerals and vitamins. Once more, this was considered a manifestation of mothers' ignorance of nutritional needs in pregnancy and lactation. "It has been found in Greece and Yugoslavia that the prolonged breast-feeding, which is the usual practice of peasant mothers, rather increases than prevents the amount of rickets in the children, showing that the diet of the nursing mother is seriously deficient."[13]

---

11 [McDougall, E.J.] "Rural dietaries," 1939, p. 474.

12 Guillem-Llobat, Perdiguero, 2006a, p. 31-40.

13 [McDougall, E.J.] "Rural dietaries," 1939, p. 474.

Please note again that criticising popular dietary habits was a widespread practice in most technical reports. Despite the availability of milk, eggs, meat and vegetables, experts accused mothers: they were unaware of how important it was to increase their intake of these foods. McDougall stated: "Amongst the slightly older children also, wrong feeding is probably more common in the country districts than in the towns, due to greater ignorance, as well as to lower purchasing power."[14]

The concern about deficiency diseases in the rural areas appeared mainly in the 1930s as a consequence of the international crisis. Not many dietary surveys could give exact figures to estimate whether the intake of vitamins and minerals was enough to meet physiological requirements, but certain signs of shortage of one or more vitamins could explain the symptoms of deficiency diseases frequently reported amongst rural populations in many parts of Europe. "Cases of night blindness and skin affections attributable to vitamin-A deficiency have been reported among rural communities in parts of Sweden, Norway, Finland, Czechoslovakia and Yugoslavia. This was seen particularly in the spring, when the diet was at its poorest."[15] Scurvy cases were soon associated by experts to vitamin C deficiencies in the diet; rickets was widespread among rural children in poor areas due to a shortage of vitamin D, calcium and fats in the diet. Lack of iodine provoked severe deficiencies, cretinism and mixoedema in the poorest areas of Extremadura, in rural Spain. Nutritional deficiencies and malnutrition were indeed a threat for the new generations, and the new science of nutrition supported by state policies posed a sort of eugenic issue.

In Muslim rural communities of Yugoslavia, with women living a secluded life, some cases of osteomalacia and osteroporosis had been reported reflecting a shortage of vitamin D and calcium in the diet and a lack of exposure to sun light. Those cases were probably even more frequent in towns than in rural districts. Pellagra cases appeared every spring in rural areas of Romania, where maize was the staple foodstuff. Once more, pellagra cases were easily avoidable; they indicated a dietary deficiency that could be prevented simply by improving dietary habits.

Foodstuffs availability in rural areas, as well as farm and agriculture production were important but, for the experts, education became the keyword, the eligible and most prominent method to change habits and subsequently improve rural standards of nutrition. Spreading scientific knowledge among the rural populations would civilise them. Now and

14 [McDougall, E.J.] "Rural dietaries," 1939, p. 474.

15 [McDougall, E.J.] "Rural dietaries," 1939, p. 474-475.

again popular culture and the experts' scientific knowledge were confronted. McDougall's report stated that: "The majority of rural housewives in Europe know little or nothing of the principles of nutrition, and they might frequently be able to feed their families more adequately if they knew the relative value of different foodstuffs."[16]

In fact, cultural habits attached to the consumption of certain foods varied considerably in different countries and regions. Milk could be considered a valuable foodstuff, being drunk by old and young, or, on the contrary, discarded for adults and only given to very young children and invalids. Some peasants did not grow vegetables for their own use while others grew and ate a variety of vegetables – even in the same or very close areas – and thereby the latter escaped the pellagra and other deficiency diseases. Experts concluded that ignorance in the rural population was a serious wastage of potential foodstuffs in rural communities that should be resolved through education. Once again, cultural habits were confronted: whey was used as pig feed or thrown away in some rural areas, while in others the peasants would take it home for cooking, adding valuable minerals to their diet. Here, the animals' blood was thrown away after slaughtering, and there the blood was made into sausages or drunk as soup.

Education was called to rationalise feeding habits and therefore help to prevent such a loss of valuable foodstuffs. "Education in the feeding of infants and growing children would also be of immense value in most villages of Europe, for it is here that ignorance is the greatest danger to health."[17] Many European countries realised the urgent need for education to change rural dietaries, and started campaigns to instruct the rural housewife, that being one of the most frequently recommended strategies.

Apart from education, in areas where peasants did not have sufficient land to produce all the foods a family needed or enough money to buy an adequate diet, planned assistance from the State was required to procure a healthy diet.

> The methods used to help the peasant must depend on the individual State. In some cases, agricultural credit is given to enable the farmer to buy equipment to increase production; in other cases, the agricultural producer may get relief from taxes, direct subsidies, family allowances, or free seed or stock from the State.[18]

---

16 [McDougall, E.J.] "Rural dietaries," 1939, p. 477.

17 [McDougall, E.J.] "Rural dietaries," 1939, p. 476.

18 [McDougall, E.J.] "Rural dietaries," 1939, p. 477.

State relief in the form of food was often given to destitute rural families during the big crisis and in war and post-war years. Rationing standards for families and individuals and the scheme for a minimum diet was also based on experts work on physiology of nutrition. Village children were sometimes given free or very cheap meals at school or in public dining rooms. Famine and malnutrition required immediate, urgent action yet, the experts agreed that "these relief measures only touch the fringe of the problem and offer no real solution."[19] The background – the economic dimension of the serious deficiencies in rural nutrition – could only be improved through agricultural and economic readjustments, both nationally and internationally. The complexity of the problem was discussed in the *Final Report of the Mixed Committee on Nutrition* (1937), which considered nutrition in relation to a wider perspective including agriculture and economic policy.[20]

The critical situation of nutrition in rural Europe during the 1930s got worse as a consequence of the Second World War. We shall devote the next chapter to discussing the negative effects of the war.

19 [McDougall, E.J.] "Rural dietaries," 1939, p. 477.

20 *Final Report*, 1937.

CHAPTER 9

Nutrition and the War

The high hopes on the science of nutrition as the nucleus of social change collapsed under the exceptional crisis posed by the Spanish Civil War and the Second World War. Both conflicts led to serious deterioration in living conditions in Europe, food availability and health status becoming main concerns with national and international organisations.[1] In the case of Spain, the benefits produced by the social and sanitary reforms introduced by the republican government since 1931 were threatened by the fascist military *coup d'état* in 1936.[2]

Nutrition problems during the Spanish Civil War

At the end of that year, the League of Nations, following a proposal by the Spanish government, adopted a resolution to send a group of experts to survey the situation. The evaluation of the nutritional state of the population and the strategy to guarantee food availability was not only a matter that impacted upon the economy and public health, but also an essential aspect in military terms that could give advantage in war. The mission was entrusted to Antoine Lasnet, medical officer and a member of the French Academy of Medicine; Dr. Jean Laigret, from the Pasteur Institute in Tunis, and Dr. C. Wroczynski, Chief Medical Adviser to the Ministry of National Education in Warsaw. At the beginning of 1937 a report was presented to the Council.[3]

The Commission paid special attention to the dietary condition of refugees, since food supply prospects in certain areas were bleak. Its report dealt with three fundamental problems: health organisation, the epidemiological situation, dietary prospects, and problems arising from the evacuation of refugees.[4]

---

1 Biraud, M., "Health in Europe. A Survey of the Epidemic and Nutritional Situation," *League of Nations Bulletin of the Health Organisation*, 1943-1944, Vol. 10, p. 557-699; Barona, 2007b.

2 Barona, 2006c and Barona, 2007b.

3 *Rapport sur la mission sanitaire en Espagne (28 décembre 1936-15 janvier 1937)*, Société des Nations, Geneva, 1937.

4 Anguera A., "Servicios sanitarios con motivo de la inmigración durante la guerra," *Revista de Sanidad e Higiene Pública*, 1938/1939, Vol. 1, p. 25-42; García Luquero,

During the first year of the war all the available data showed a controlled epidemiological situation without signs of degradation. There were no unexpected epidemic outbreaks. The health of the population in the republican zone remained within usual limits. The stable population had enough supplies, but there were severe shortages among the refugees. This apparent normality was a surprise for the League of Nations experts visiting Spain at the beginning of 1937. But the situation began to worsen, as shown by the evolution of the general mortality rate. During 1930-1935 the rate was 14.5 per thousand, and in 1937 it was only 15.5. But the rate increased gradually during the war reaching a peak of 19.2 per thousand in 1938. When the civil war finished, there was a decrease in general mortality for a three-month period but in 1940 an increase brought the rate up to 16.6 per thousand. 1941 showed a new increase due, in part, to food shortages and to the high infant mortality subsequent to the spectacular birth rise in 1940.[5]

The system of epidemiological data collection put in place by Marcelino Pascua[6] during the first republican biennium had been profoundly altered by the war and the collection of data was imperfect. Yet, it still permitted the identification of the four principal problems that required attention, that is, typhoid fever, spotted fever, smallpox, and bacillary dysentery. All of them were logical and inevitable problems, given the living conditions during the war.[7]

According to the League of Nations' 1937 report, typhoid fever had been an endemic problem before the war due to poor hygiene in water for human consumption. The number of cases at the start of the 1920s oscillated between 15,000 and 20,000 annually, provoking from 3,000 to 4,000 deaths. During 1934-1935 the number of cases was strongly reduced. But the situation worsened from the start of the war due to the deterioration of sanitary conditions and the movement of refugees, as shown by the data employed by the expert committee, originally from statistics compiled by the National Hospital of Infectious Diseases. In the second half of 1936 there were 358 cases, 42 of which ending in death. At any rate, the experts expressed their reserve and thought that health services had reorganised and that bacteriological water testing

---

"Aspectos sanitarios de la evacuación de refugiados en Santander," *Revista de Sanidad e Higiene Pública*, 1938-1939, Vol. 1, p. 68-81.

5 Barona, 2007b.

6 Marcelino Pascua was a former fellow of the Rockefeller Foundation at the Johns Hopkins School of Public Health and General Director for Health in the socialist government 1931-1933. After the war he went to the exile becoming head of the statistics office of the World Health Organisation.

7 *Rapport sur la mission sanitaire*, 1937, p. 72-73.

was being carried out on a regular basis. There was no fear of an epidemic, and therefore, an intensification of typhoid vaccination was not recommended.

Spotted fever, traditionally associated with situations of war or catastrophe, had not yet shown signs of exacerbation at the start of 1937, when the experts from the League of Nations wrote their report. It had been a serious problem in Spain in 1919 and 1920, but had been brought under control in 1935.[8] The commission experts were satisfied with the measures put into place by Spanish authorities: immediate de-lousing and vaccination if there was potential for an epidemic.

Bacillary dysentery had caused 64 deaths in 1934 and 105 deaths in 1935, worsening being feared at the start of the war. As a consequence, a special coprological examination service was established at the *Instituto Nacional de Higiene*, which continued until November 1937.[9] Only eight cases and one death were recorded, but there were many cases in Asturias, although exact numbers could not be estimated. The experts did not consider the situation to be epidemic. All the surveillance systems were in place in case the problem worsened.

Other health problems were deemed to be of less importance or unaffected by war conditions. There were no deaths caused by smallpox, although experts recommended that medical authorities be on the alert for deaths from smallpox in Spanish Morocco and Portugal. The health mission did not notice a worsening in the morbidity or in malarial mortality, and other infectious diseases had not been affected by the war. The *hospitales de carabineros*, new institutions founded in the frame of the new war health care system had the control of malaria as their main target.[10]

Compiled by the *Hospital Nacional de Enfermedades Infecciosas*, the official data on diseases which required notification, relative to the area of Madrid during the period 19 July 1936 - 1 January 1937 were as follows:

---

8 It caused 227 and 153 deaths respectively. Only three deaths in 1935.

9 *Rapport sur la mission sanitaire*, 1937, p. 73-74.

10 Calandre, C., "El Dr. Luis Calandre Ibáñez. Su actuación en la Guerra Civil Española (1937-1939)," *Frente de Madrid*, 2007, Vol. 11, p. 6-11.

Diseases in the area of Madrid, 19 July 1936 - 1 January 1937

	Cases	Deaths	Lethality %
Typhoid Fever	358	42	11.7
Paratyphoid Fever	6	--	--
Pneumonia	88	9	10.2
Dysentery	8	1	12.5
Puerperal septicaemia	10	6	60
Tetanus	5	2	40
Pertussis	83	3	3.6
Poliomyelitis	1	--	--
Malaria	46	--	--
Diphteria	3	--	--
Anthrax	15	--	--
Tuberculous Meningitis	14	14	100
Malta Fever	20	2	10
Scarlet Fever	80	8	10
Erysipelas	71	4	5.6
Brain-Spinal Meningitis	4	2	50
Rubella	99	10	10
Lung Tuberculosis	456	58	12.3
Carbuncle	8	--	--
Endocarditis	26	8	30
Encephalitis	1	1	100
Flue	41	2	1.8
Chickenpox	11	--	--
Tonsillitis	30	--	--
Other cases	287	40	15
Total	1,778	212	11.9

The report also included data compiled in Valencia for all the republican zones, but for only three weeks in December. From this data, the 258 cases of typhoid fever are to be noted, with 42 deaths, in addition to the incidence of German measles, with 1,027 cases, but only 4 deaths.

The whole of the epidemiological survey did not detect the appearance of epidemic or even sporadic outbreaks. The measures adopted by the republican government in this matter consisted of recruiting all the medical professionals of the country, coordinating the actions of the civil and military medical authorities, adopting special measures to ensure the proper functioning of medical aid on the front and developing a vaccination campaign. There was typhoid and paratyphoid fever vaccination in the army, and a rather widespread paratyphoid fever vaccination existed among the civilian population. Smallpox vaccination was compulsory, yet vaccination against diphtheria was rare, given that this measure had never been that widespread among the population. There was no other type of preventive vaccination applied to soldiers, not even against tetanus.

From their observations and the official data compiled, the League of Nations experts considered the health situation to be satisfactory at the start of 1937, although they feared the spread of typhoid and spotted fevers. They therefore recommended compulsory vaccination, and water and food testing. With regard to spotted fever, they laid out recommendations for the improvement of treatment and prevention that included the use of portable de-lousing devices and treatment material, general immunisation against typhus for health workers and improving the availability of vaccines. They thought it necessary to outfit municipal and provincial centres with specific areas for the treatment of patients with infectious diseases, to provide disinfection devices for health services, these being clearly inadequate; to isolate contagious patients and improve the system of epidemiological data collection in order to detect any sign of deterioration in the sanitary situation at any time. A central point was the training of doctors specialised in epidemics; these could be specifically assigned to prophylaxis and the fight against infections and be incorporated into asylums, prisons and other places where large groups of people lived.

The report presented by J. A. Palanca to the League of Nations in 1939 on the Francoist side commented the main health problems in the rebel Army but also the health situation of the civil population.[11] The report was rather unrealistic in trying to show that the actions taken before the war allowed a controlled epidemiological situation during the war in the Francoist zone. Palanca, in a triumphant tone, mentioned that widespread use of the typhoid vaccination along with strict water testing had prevented any problems. The efforts had to be redoubled when the Northern provinces were taken (Santander, Vizcaya, Asturias) but, according to his testimony, the situation remained under control. He even stated that mortality due to disease probably continued to decrease throughout the war. He also cited the good situation with respect to spotted fever, arguing that there had only been one case on the Francoist side despite the large contingents of refugees that came from the enemy zone. The incessant taking over of new territory had required the special

---

11 Palanca y Martínez Fortún, J. A. *Les services sanitaires espagnols pendant la guerre civile*, Genève, Societé de Nations, 1939. Palanca was a conservative hygienist belonging to the group of experts in public health leading reforms in Spain during the previous decade; he was an intern of the Rockefeller Foundation. After the start of the Civil War he became the head of health politics in francoist, nationalist side.

surveillance of ports, prisons, asylums and concentration camps. A real *cordon sanitaire* had been established with disinfection cabinets and delousing stations in areas of contact with the enemy in order to prevent the disease.

With regard to malaria, Palanca's report indicated that the anti-malarial programme was, as far as possible, ongoing, as per the anti-malaria campaigns implemented before the war, and that the medical dispensaries functioned with regularity, having sufficient medication.[12] But the possible exacerbation of the disease was recognised. The movements of the troops and the destruction of the cities had given way to new malarial outbreaks that needed to be examined, especially in areas where anopheles existed without malaria cases. Although there were no figures, it was thought that the number of malaria patients, especially in the armies of both sides, must have been considerable.

Palanca briefly mentioned leprosy in order to point out that the same policy of patient isolation that had existed before the war was being followed, using the available institutions in Galicia and Andalusia. Medication was sufficient, and with the end of the war, the leper colony of Fontilles was available once again to isolate the patients.

On the other hand, venereal diseases were a serious problem, as usual during wartime, particularly among soldiers. Outpatient treatment at anti-venereal dispensaries continued, as well as the reserving of some isolation beds in hospitals and the creation of a few isolation centres for those patients. In addition, prostitutes who were contagious were isolated. Medication in the form of arsenic and bismuth was the therapeutic weapon that was used to stop the problem.

One of the problems that Palanca recognised as being of greater seriousness was that of diphtheria, whose mortality rate had decreased to 5 per 100,000 inhabitants in 1935. The war had not seemed to worsen this figure, but the number of cases had increased. Anatoxin had not been available due to the fact that heat cabinets were being used for the production of the typhoid vaccine. The situation was turned around, thanks to some provincial laboratories that were producing anatoxin and also to the production of antidiphtheria serum, which would help in the treatment of the disease.

The report showed some concern with respect to smallpox since the number of cases had increased and various epidemic outbreaks that were difficult to isolate had appeared due to the problems associated with transport. An intensive vaccination campaign was being undertaken and the sanitary institutions produced "millions of doses of the vaccine,"

---

12 Palanca y Martínez Fortún, 1939.

despite some technical difficulties. At any rate, mortality was nil since the majority of the cases were caused by varioloid and in the few cases of smallpox there had been no complications.

Although Palanca was also somewhat concerned with other problems such as trichinosis and rabies, aggravated by difficulties in veterinary care, he believed them to be under control once surveillance and treatment programmes were reinstated. The completion of Palanca's report coincided with the end of the war, a time at which the necessary reconstruction of health care to the population was already underway.[13]

The evacuation of the refugees fleeing from the front to neighbouring areas was a fundamental aspect regarding the health of the population. The report of the League of Nations showed that 250,000 refugees from Extremadura lived in Jaén, Ciudad Real and Toledo; and Catalonia had received a large quantity of refugees from Aragón. The flow of refugees aroused the spontaneous solidarity of the families living in the hosting zones, but there was a need to set up a National Committee for War Refugees. The provincial and local delegations of this committee were in charge of the evacuation, distribution and fostering of the refugees.[14] The money for the care of the refugees came from private sources and the national budget.

The magnitude of the problems raised by the evacuation of the population from the front was enormous. At the end of 1936 they accounted for more than one million. Of them, 350,000 were fostered in Catalonia and 250,000 in Valencia.[15] The refugees accounted for 14% of the whole population of the country. The capacity to foster new refugees was on the verge of saturation, and food shortage began in some areas. The evacuation of the capital, Madrid, under siege, was very hard and the experts predicted a dramatic worsening of the health and nutritional status of the population.

The Commission paid special attention to the dietary condition of refugees, since food supply prospects in certain areas were bleak. Its report dealt with three fundamental problems: health organisation, epidemiological situation, dietary prospects, and problems arising from the evacuation of refugees. Food supplies became a problem affecting more than 1,200,000 inhabitants during the siege of Madrid. It became worse with more than 300,000 refugees during the first months of the war.

---

13 Palanca y Martínez Fortún, 1939.

14 *Rapport sur la mission sanitaire*, 1937, p. 73-74.

15 *Rapport sur la mission sanitaire*, 1937, p. 86.

The military front divided the country into two sides. The east was under Republican control and the rebels took the west and the north. The Republican zone produced wheat, rice, vegetables, fruits, and wine. The area controlled by Franco's troops produced cereals but mainly for grazing.[16] The experts from the League of Nations predicted that the inhabitants of Madrid would go short of meat and milk. The supply of flour, olive oil, fruits, pulses, and vegetables was guaranteed if the republican authorities were able to defend the transport infrastructure. Although the lack of milk and meat was alleviated by other products, transport difficulties meant long queues of people.[17]

As from the second half of 1937, severe food problems hit the Spanish population, comparatively worse than the shortages in central Europe during the First World War.[18] Madrid saw a decrease in the caloric value of its diet as compared with the first winter of the war, and this led to nutritional deficiencies and progressive malnutrition in the whole population.[19]

The state of war changed the social and political dimension of food availability and nutrition, which now became a military tool. Following international recommendations, the Spanish Government established an *Instituto Nacional de Higiene de la Alimentación* [National Institute for Food Hygiene], where experts in physiology of nutrition aimed to coordinate nutritional policies both for the civil population and the military forces under the direction of José Puche, Professor of physiology at the University of Valencia and expert on nutrition. They Spanish experts knew about the latest developments in nutrition physiology and the research work discussed and published by the technical committee of the League of Nations.[20] As from January 1937, scientific criteria were used to implement a system on the basis of family or personal food rationing and special norms for ill people.[21] Single rations included

16 *Rapport sur la mission sanitaire*, 1937.

17 *Rapport sur la mission sanitaire*, 1937.

18 *Rapport sur la mission sanitaire*, 1937.

19 Grande Covián, F., *La alimentación en Madrid durante la Guerra. (Estudio de la dieta suministrada a la población civil madrileña durante diecinueve meses de guerra: Agosto 1937 a Febrero 1939)*, Publicación de la Revista de Sanidad e Higiene Pública, 1939.

20 The Technical Commission on Nutrition was chaired in March 1937 by Edward Mellanby, and composed by sixteen members. Teófilo Hernando, a Professor of Pharmacology in Madrid, Enrique Suñer, a Professor of Pediatry and José Murillo, director of the Spanish Institute for Food and Medicines were Spanish representatives.

21 Jiménez García, F., Grande Covián, F., "Sobre los trastornos carenciales observados en Madrid durante la Guerra. I. Los cuadros clínicos presentados con más frecuencia

150 grams of fresh or tinned meat, which could be replaced by 100 grams of ham, 200 grams of fresh fish, 100 grams of preserved fish or 80 grams of codfish; dairy products: half a litre of fresh milk, 130 grams of condensed milk, 200 grams of concentrated milk or 75 grams of cheese; a quarter of a litre of olive oil, 200 grams of butter or 100 grams of bacon; 250 grams of potatoes or 100 grams of lentils, 150 of dry string beans, 180 grams of rice, 150 grams of wide string beans or 100 grams of dry chickpeas; 150 grams of fresh vegetables or 500 grams of preserved fruit or vegetables (tomatoes, etc.); 25 grams of coffee or tea, or 30 grams of chocolate or 50 grams of coconut; 50 grams of sugar or 80 grams of honey, and half a kilo of bread.

At the beginning of 1937, Spanish health officers advised that the demand of basic products had almost been covered by the domestic agricultural produce. Nevertheless, in anticipation of future shortages, 120 tons of potatoes were imported from Holland. The main problem, however, was a deficiency of transport. In 1937 the food supply had not yet led to critical problems of hunger, deficiency diseases, or malnutrition, but experts expressed their concern: "If we consider the hundreds of thousands of women and children who live in Madrid, we can only conclude that it will be necessary to evacuate them as soon as possible… as food deficiency is a big threat."[22]

Nutrition had become central to the war. In mid-1939, the Technical Commission on Nutrition of the League of Nations presented a report of the work done between June 1938 and April 1939, including a section on the critical situation of the feeding of refugees in Spain and the need to take emergency measures to avoid starvation:

> […] During its August session, the attention of the Special Committee was drawn to the fact that, even in Europe, disturbing conditions existed in which the problem was no longer to lay down the bases for a satisfactory diet, but rather to prevent the population from dying from starvation. This was, more particularly, the position of Spain, and, to cope with it, the Society of Friends sought guidance in the preparation of an emergency diet for the refugees.
>
> The Committee suggested a diet of this character. It is composed of whole wheat, brewer's dried yeast, cod-liver oil and various salts, and is so designed as to include vitamins and essential inorganic constituents. At the same time, the Committee pointed out that such a diet was at most adequate

y su clasificación," *Revista Clínica Española*, 1940a, Vol. 1, p. 313-318; Jiménez García, F., Grande Covián, F., "Algunas observaciones sobre las dietas consumidas por los enfermos carenciales de Madrid," *Revista Clínica Española*, 1940b, Vol. 1, No. 1.

22 *Rapport sur la mission sanitaire*, 1937, p. 89.

to sustain life and to prevent the appearance, during a limited period, of the more serious effects of malnutrition. It could only be looked upon as an emergency diet, to be supplemented at the earliest possible moment by fresh foods."[23]

From November 1936, as a result of the siege of the city by rebel troops, a period of dietary restrictions started for the people of Madrid, worsening over time and finally affecting the majority of citizens. The City Council introduced a *Family supply card* and put a ban on the free traffic of foodstuffs. As a consequence, most of the inhabitants were given the same ration for much of the war and Madrid's society was turned into a laboratory to analyse the effects of a prolonged lack of food, since the period of famine and scarcity lasted more than two years. A group of experts from the National Institute of Food Hygiene completed a study of the diet of Madrid's population during the nineteen-month siege, from August 1937 to February 1939. F. Grande Covian published a synthesis of the results.[24]

The average calorie value of the diets provided during the nineteen-month period came to 1,060 calories a day, representing 49.7% of the minimum acceptable level. In the last year of the war, the average was 944 calories, that is, 43.3% of the minimum daily intake. The calorie value of the diet dropped steadily, from 1,514 daily calories in August 1937 to 852 in February 1939, a leap downward from 70% to 36% of the minimum diet. From an energy point of view, it was definitely a poor diet; besides, the main foodstuffs were bread, oil, rice, legumes and sugar, animal products accounting for just 4.7% of the total calorie value. While the approximate protein need was estimated at 60 grams per day, the average figure for the nineteen months was 34 grams, i.e. 56% lower. In fact, the diet on the *Cartilla de Racionamiento* represented an average value of 25 grams per day.[25]

The diet was deficient in fats (41% of the minimum diet) and carbohydrates (53% of the minimum daily intake) but also in minerals and vitamins. Group A and C vitamins were below the minimum threshold, group B ones showed a high deficit, and only the good weather of the city made up for the shortage of vitamin D. All these data placed the population of Madrid in a more negative position than the German population during the First World War, whose calorie coefficient ranged between 1,400 and 1,800 calories per person per day.

---

23 "Report on the work of the Health Organisation," 1939, p. 32.

24 Grande Covián, 1939.

25 Grande Covián, 1939, p. 45-46.

In the study of deficiency diseases associated to malnutrition, the Spanish experts F. Jiménez and F. Grande Covián estimated the average caloric value of the diet of the Madrid population to be 2,130 calories daily before the war. In August 1937 that figure had been halved.[26] The feeding of the population reached a critical point in October 1938 when only 150 grams of bread by person could be allocated and the daily diet of a great deal of the population was limited to a cup of Malta coffee with or without sugar for breakfast; a plate of lentil soup with a little bread for lunch, and some rice with a little bread for dinner. That type of diet only contributed between 800 and 1000 calories and caused a very significant loss in body weight. Surveys developed by nutritionists at the end of the war indicated that the average loss of weight of the population in Madrid as a result of deficiency diseases represented approximately 30% of their weight before the start of the war.[27]

The new science of nutrition was useful in identifying the problems but was impotent in offering practical solutions. The Spanish group of experts began to detect simple or non-specific malnutrition and several deficiency diseases, which attracted the attention of physiologists, nutritionists and clinicians. There were neither reliable nor comprehensive statistics. Only data on mortality in the first year of the war were available, but they were inaccurate due to an inefficient system of recording epidemiological data. From the research published by nutritional experts we know that the main deficiency illnesses in Madrid were pellagra, "pellagra sine pellagra," deficiency neuropathies, optic and acoustic neuritis, simple glossitis, and hunger oedema.[28] Most of these conditions were associated with avitaminoses or with a deficiency of proteins and became worse during the post-war period.[29]

During the early 1940s Francisco Jiménez García and Francisco Grande Covián, from the *Instituto Nacional de Higiene de la Alimentación* in Madrid, published a series of research articles in the *Revista Clínica Española* including plenty of records on the deficiency illnesses suffered by the inhabitants of Madrid during the war and the

---

26 Jiménez García, F., Grande Covián, F., "Sobre los trastornos carenciales observados en Madrid durante la Guerra. I. Los cuadros clínicos presentados con más frecuencia y su clasificación," *Revista Clínica Española*, 1, (1940a), p. 313-318; Jiménez García, F., Grande Covián, F., "Algunas observaciones sobre las dietas consumidas por los enfermos carenciales de Madrid," *Revista Clinica Española*, I(1), (1940b).

27 Jiménez García, Grande Covián, 1940a, p. 313-318; Jiménez García, Grande Covián, 1940b.

28 For a broader analysis see Barona, Perdiguero, 2007.

29 García-Albea Ristol E., "Las neuropatías carenciales en Madrid durante la Guerra Civil," *Neurología*, 1999, Vol. 14, p. 122-129.

early post-war period.[30] Despite the dramatic nutritional status of the population, avitaminoses A, C and D were very infrequent, exceptionally causing haemeralopia, scurvy and rickets. Around 1943 and 1944 deficiency illnesses similar to the ones described in Madrid began to appear among the population of some European countries as a consequence of the Second World War.[31]

The situation of the Spanish population hardly improved during the first years after the conflict. In fact, in several ways, the nutritional status of the Spanish population worsened during the post-war period, as reflected in 1943 by Yves Biraud, an expert form the League of Nations, in his assessment of nutrition in Europe.[32]

Once the war had ended, Palanca, fully responsible for public health organisation and policies following Franco's victory, presented a new report on the health situation in Spain,[33] a report that appeared to be more pessimistic than the previous one, which had tried to transmit the idea of a controlled and reorganised response to all the problems that had arisen during the war. That is why he thought that during 1939 there had been changes and the epidemiological situation had worsened since the end of the war. Nevertheless, he did not hasten to point out that this trend was not evolving catastrophically, thanks to the effort of health workers of the Directorate General of Public Health.

The changes that Palanca was referring to were the reappearance of some cases of spotted fever and smallpox which even led to small outbreaks in certain provinces. Francoist health authorities blamed smallpox propagation on the large cross-country movements of people at the end of the war, both military and civilian. Nevertheless, they remained optimistic since in his opinion this apparent propagation did not reflect reality given that in the majority of provinces, infectious cases had run into a barrier of immunised persons, definitively detaining the spread of the disease.

Spotted fever, which according to Palanca's report had not produced any cases in the country prior to contact with the enemy lines, started to appear in the province of Cuenca, where a small outbreak took place. The origin of the epidemic was related to cases that had appeared in the province of Murcia prior to its conquest by fascist troops. A similar cause was to blame for the cases reported in Malaga, Madrid and a small

---

30 This research has been partially analysed by Del Cura, Huertas García-Alejo, 2006, p. 50-89; Barona, 2007b, p. 31-34; Garcia-Albea Ristol, 1999, p. 122-129.

31 Barona, 2007b.

32 Biraud, 1943/1944.

33 Palanca y Martínez Fortún, 1939, p. 40-52.

outbreak that had recently occurred in Villarrobledo (Albacete). The origin of the disease was always attributed to the republican area and the report tried to minimise its importance.

Palanca pointed out that the deficient health conditions after the war that had been worsened by the large movements of the population had reached their peak in Madrid. During a period of two years and a half the city had been subject to an incomplete siege and as a consequence, the population had lived under really poor provisioning and housing conditions. In addition to this, in the post-war period, Madrid's privileged central location made it subject to population movements, both of immigrants and emigrants, as well as a constant influx and efflux of masses of people in transit. As a result, there appeared cases of spotted fever and smallpox in the capital and an unprecedented number of cases of diphtheria and a notable worsening of endemic typhoid fever.

With regard to smallpox, the situation worsened in the final year of the war. Data were most significant; from there being practically no reported cases before November 1938 to a total of 288 official cases in ten months, even though the real occurrence of the disease must have been even greater. The end of the vaccination policies was the reason behind this worsening, since the majority of the cases appeared in population groups that had not been vaccinated or that had been vaccinated more than seven years before.

Diphtheria started to provoke new cases from August 1938. In Madrid 254 cases were reported in September, with 27 deaths, which prompted emergency measures for the production of anti-diphtheria serum and anatoxin vaccination campaigns. But at the end of 1939, diphtheria continued to rise among children.

Finally, typhoid fever constituted the other cause of death for the Spanish population at the end of the civil war, provoking epidemic situations in many towns, with processes of re-infection that were very difficult to control. A strategy was developed to isolate patients in hospitals, this being difficult to apply, as was the chimerical disinfection of instruments and products that could potentially transmit the disease, as well as vaccination campaigns: more than three hundred thousand vaccinations were administered in a few months. But medical technology could hardly palliate the great health problems that were caused by destitution. The ravages of a three-year civil war and the consequences of poverty during the post-war period placed Spanish society, at the start of the 1940s, in a greatly deteriorated social and health situation.

We can turn to still another source to help us evaluate the health condition of the Spanish population at the end of the war. On August 20th, 1939 the Rockefeller Foundation drew up a report on the situation of the

Spanish society with data from several aspects of Spanish life. Speaking about health, the report recognized the achievements of the republican health services but pointed out the epidemic outbreaks and the appearance of malnutrition in wide sectors of the population.[34]

The report recognised that before the war, starting from a nucleus mainly composed of old interns from the Rockefeller Foundation, there had been great progress in the health organisation. But the report stated that the situation deteriorated after 1939 and, immediately after the war epidemic diseases appeared. It reported on the increased prevalence of smallpox, spotted fever, malaria and typhoid fever, even though the spread of the latter was not yet considered alarming.

The report also noted the destruction of sanitary equipment in Madrid, where many centres located on the firing line had been reduced to rubble. The destruction had also been quite serious in the rest of the country, various provincial hygiene institutes – cornerstones of the territorial health organisation – having been seriously damaged. The Foundation was aware that an important task of reconstruction had to be carried out in a very complex situation. Indeed, the government was in the middle of serious financial difficulties. The cost of war had been enormous, the reserves of gold had disappeared and the cost of living in Madrid had doubled, inflation had risen to unprecedented extremes and the taxation system still lacked a solid foundation. A significant part of Madrid had been destroyed and an incalculable number of towns and cities had been reduced to rubble. In addition to those who had lost their lives, wide sectors of the population had become immersed in poverty. The report considered that the State was making great strides to help those affected, but it also had to face this terrible situation in an international context of isolation and conflict.

But probably the most striking aspect of the report was its positive attitude towards the new health authorities and especially the Director General for Health, J.A. Palanca. It stated that, except in some cases, the medical workers had continued working during the strife, respected by both fronts as experts, whose work had no reason to be interfered with. The process of purging the public health workers that had worked in the "red" zone was underway, but nevertheless the Rockefeller Foundation predicted a happy ending.[35] Of course, the information that the Rockefeller Foundation received was manipulated and did not correspond to

[34] Rockefeller Foundation, *Report on the health situation in Spain*, 20 August, 1939. Rockefeller Archive Centre, New York. See also the 'Notes on the food situation in Spain" drawn up on October 1940 by F. H. Janey from the Rockefeller Foundation.

[35] A whole chapter in Barona, Bernabeu, 2008 is devoted to show the great handicap caused by the exile of public health experts.

reality, given that the public health experts were gravely punished after the war and the majority went into exile and in the following decades participated actively in foreign and international posts in Venezuela, Mexico, Cuba, the Pan-American Health Office or in the World Health Organisation.[36]

Because of the Second World War and the international isolation of Franco's government, the situation of the Spanish population hardly improved during the first years after the conflict. In fact, in several ways, the nutritional status of the Spanish population worsened during those years, as was reflected in Spanish medical reports.

The consequences of the Second World War

An evaluation of the nutritional problems in Europe as a consequence of the war was required, but a complete and accurate study of its influence on the impairment of public health was not possible until some time after the end of the hostilities. Nevertheless, health authorities and relief Organisations needed any helpful information to overcome the hard wartime situation as regards both nutrition and epidemics. Two principal reports were made public in 1943 by the Health Organisation of the League of Nations. One of them was published under the title "Health in Europe" by Yves M. Biraud, the Head of the Service of Epidemiological Intelligence and Public Health Statistics of the League of Nations.[37] The second was a technical report on "Famine disease and its treatment in internment camps." Both offered a terrible picture to the health and nutritional situation in Europe during the early 1940s.

Biraud's report was preceded by a series of articles in the medical literature pointing out "the shortcomings of rationing, losses of weight of children and adults; increase in the incidence of certain communicable diseases; changes in the prevalence and character of tuberculosis; the increase in both infant and general death rates."[38] In spite the usefulness of those partial approaches, no comprehensive study had been published based on a large body of statistical material and therefore his aim was to furnish the statistical materials collected from many reports at the Service of Epidemiological Intelligence and Public health Statistics of the League of Nations in Geneva. Biraud was aware of the limitations of those records, which did not cover adequately countries like Poland or Greece which had suffered most from nutritional deficiencies and famine. The make-up and size of populations and cities in many

---

36 Barona, Bernabeu, 2008.

37 Biraud, 1943-1944.

38 Biraud, 1943-1944, p. 559.

European countries were deeply altered by enrolment in the forces, migrations of refugees, deportations, attraction to war industries and evacuations, thus making it difficult for death rates to be satisfactory.

But Biraud's memorandum was accurate enough to give an adequate approach to the trend of health impairment in Europe in 1943. Divergence in the trends of general mortality in different countries gave a measure of the influence of insufficient feeding. Although the main target was to report the health situation as a consequence of the war, the author aimed to "give a measure of the influence of insufficient feeding."[39]

> To estimate the food situation in Europe, we have made use of: a) computations concerning normal consumption of staple foods in European countries based on documents issued by the Economic Intelligence Service of the League, and documents on war-time rationing and consumption published by the same Service; b) a series of monographs published in 1939 for the European Conference on Rural life, which cover the agricultural situation in European countries; c) data on food restrictions, taken from the daily press, medical periodicals, and private studies; and d) reports from national health administrations and from relief organisations, both official and private.[40]

Biraud's attempt to make a preliminary estimate of the health and nutritional situation of the European population could benefit from the experience gained in the study of the consequences of the First World War and the economic depression upon public health. In the absence of any synthetic index reflecting the state of health of a population, recourse to morbidity and mortality rates was the best approach, since representing "the amount of sickness and of death, express, as it were, the reverse of health."[41] Moreover morbidity records for the war period were seldom available, army medical statistics were not made public and in war time workers were less likely to absent themselves from work on account of minor ailments or fatigue than they would be under normal circumstances. The change of occupation to war industries falsified any attempt of comparison between rates related to working population and medical statistics concerning school children were scarcely satisfactory due to massive evacuation campaigns.

In spite of the methodological limitations due to the exceptional circumstances of the war and the scarcity of reliable records, Biraud offers a convincing landscape of the nutritional situation of most European countries. According to his memorandum, food availability in Poland

---

39 Biraud, 1943-1944, p. 561.

40 Biraud, 1943-1944, p. 561-562.

41 Biraud, 1943-1944, p. 563.

had varied enormously depending on places and social circumstances, ranging from practical sufficiency in some agricultural areas to acute shortage in cities and famine in ghettos. The effects on health were different: from mere deficiency diseases such as rickets to mass starvation. In 1943 relief efforts had been greatly reduced due to the opposition of the German occupation forces, chiefly concentrating on children.

In the Balkan region there were also considerable local differences in the effects of the food shortage, something fairly general in the south west side of the region. The situation for the USSR was not better in the absence of reliable vital statistics, especially considering the negative effects of the German seizure of a large part of its most fertile agricultural land, including the whole black-earth area.[42] The situation of the besieged population of Leningrad was dramatic, and millions of refugees had been evacuated from the war zone. According to Biraud, "[...] The hugeness of the food stores sent to the USSR under lend-lease agreements is an indication of the extent of the need."[43]

Special reference was made to the food shortage in post-war Spain:

> There food shortage was severe during the civil war in a large part of the country, indeed acute for two winters in Madrid and among the large number of prisoners. The economic and social consequences of the civil war were prolonged and aggravated by the European war, so that in 1941 the serious nature of the nutritional situation of the country appeared to be second only of that of Greece. Improvement has since taken place."[44]

During the early 1940s actual famine and resulting starvation had occurred in many population groups across Europe: inmates in internment camps, prisoners of war camps, Jews in ghettos, civil population and soldiers of besieged cities, patients in hospitals and prisoners. A considerable loss of weight and deficiency diseases had been detected among great numbers of people in cities of occupied countries, but the lack of food had been nowhere as intense and general on a nation-wide scale as it had been in Greece. Even in the peacetime period previous to the war, only a small portion of the staple foods needed to meet the population's dietary requirements were grown, according to official records. "Invasion, the cutting-off of outside supplies and large-scale requisitioning resulted in actual famine during the winter of 1941/42."[45] Famine affected the towns first and then extended to the countryside. The situation became much worse in 1943 and 1944 due to the negative

42 Biraud, 1943-1944, p. 694.

43 Biraud, 1943-1944, p. 694.

44 Biraud, 1943-1944, p. 694.

45 Biraud, 1943-1944, p. 695.

effects of inflation. In addition, the limited relief supplies allowed to enter the country were insufficient and could hardly transform the extended famine condition into a situation of chronic and severe shortage.

In its milder but chronic form, food insufficiency was considered to have caused a definite increase in tuberculosis mortality and in the general mortality rates of several countries. It was the main cause of many deaths, but also an effective contributory cause to a much greater number, particularly among elderly people and certain population groups living under exceptional circumstances.

As far as mortality is concerned, rates indicated that infants had been spared, generally speaking, although they suffered from many forms of non-fatal malnutrition, as many adults did. Stunted growth in the young was equivalent to the loss of weight in older individuals. On the other hand, food shortage and malnutrition prevailed far more severely in cities than in rural areas, a fact showing capital importance for planning food relief. Prospects were uncertain for a prompt and adequate relief which – if followed by rapid economic improvement – would result in a comparatively rapid physical rehabilitation of population groups suffering from malnutrition, with a quick fall of tuberculosis mortality rates. Experience gained during the aftermath of the First World War reinforced this perspective.

But the health situation at the end of the Second World War was not optimistic. Increased contacts due to community life and migrations resulted in a fairly marked rise in diphtheria, scarlet fever and meningitis in central, Northern and Western Europe. A similar effect was caused by typhus fever in Eastern and South-Eastern Europe. Destitution in terms of lack of food, soap, home and body linen, had contributed to the increase in typhus fever in endemic areas and among prisoners and inmates of relief institutions. However, those epidemics did not influence the incidence or severity of traditional and other epidemic diseases at the end of the war. Probably typhus fever was a threat, since its prevalence in Eastern and South-Eastern countries of Europe could be the origin of a breakdown eventually extended to other regions by troops coming from those areas, as well as from North Africa.

Biraud tried to fight exaggerated fears in the public opinion and medical professionals regarding the expansion of epidemic diseases during and after the war. The diseases causing the heaviest losses in the past had been mostly controlled: typhus fever, smallpox, enteric fever, malaria. After the Great War rural populations in Russia had a low degree of acquired immunity to common infectious diseases and migrations contributed to spreading contagion and epidemics.

> Now the epidemic situation differs considerably from what it was in 1918, as does the distribution in Europe of prisoners-of-war and refugees who will require repatriation during the armistice period. Most of them are at present in Germany, where no one of the pestilential diseases prevails (at any rate in endemic form), where malaria and other sub-tropical endemic infections are practically non-exitstant, where the population is itself practically free from lice, and where the essential rules of sanitation are generally enforced.[46]

According to this, the danger of dissemination of infection under the circumstances in 1945 was infinitely smaller than it was in 1919. A general action was in preparation. The United Nations' Relief and Rehabilitation Administration had benefited from the pioneer work of the Inter-Allied Relief Committees in London as well as national health administrations to prepare plans for repatriation of refugees and prisoners, medial relief and the fight against epidemics. National Red Cross Societies were also prepared for emergencies, and a collaborative commitment of health and statistical authorities from different countries with the Epidemiological Intelligence Service of the League of Nations was expected to face epidemic diseases and keep health administrations and relief organisations informed. Some confidence in the future capacity to get over the post-war and improve health standards after the close of the hostilities emerged from Biraud's survey.

---

46 Biraud, 1943-1944, p. 696.

CHAPTER 10

Famine Disease in Internment Camps

Internment camps were large detention centres created to confine selected groups of the population, usually for political reasons and without legal judicial trials. They usually consisted of barracks, huts, or tents, surrounded by watch towers, and contained by barbed wire fencing. In Germany, the Nazi regime established concentration camps after reaching power in 1933, and during the Second World War camps increased in size and number in many areas of Europe. Inmates came from every occupied country and others were transported from different areas. Early in 1942 the *Wirtschafts-Verwaltungshauptamt*, the Central Office for Economy and Administration of the SS, assumed operational control of the camps, and inmates were frequently worked to death as forced labourers in industrial production. They were also used as subjects for medical experiments.[1]

The nutritional situation of inmates in interment camps during the war years was a descent to hell. A report about the health condition of inmates in those institutions was published at the *League of Nations Bulletin of the Health Organisation* in 1944.[2] The memorandum was received for publication in August 1943 and reflected the work of one year of clinical research. According to the figures in the memorandum, internment camps investigated harboured some 20,000 adolescents and adult internees in 1943. The published report focused on medical aspects related to the state of health of the confined population, excluding any reference to living conditions, human rights or internal rules that could incriminate authorities. The research was published as an *anonymous* report. The work done was justified for the scientific interest and experimental value of the observations, and the practical application of the results in communities suffering from famine. The names of the doctors participating in the research were suppressed, as well as those of the internees and any geographical references of the camps.

1 Weindling, P.J., *Nazi Medicine and the Nuremberg Trials: From Medical War Crimes to Informed Consent*, New York, Palgrave Macmillan.

2 "Famine Disease and its Treatment in Internment Camps," *League of Nations Bulletin of the Health Organisation*, 1943-1944, Vol. 10, p. 722-772.

Between 1940 and 1943, the internment camps received a strong influx of inmates the number and composition of which was variable. Internees showed surprising physical and moral resistance to the very negative health and nutritional conditions to which they were submitted. The situation changed completely 12 to 16 months after the internment of about 20,000 inmates. A first outbreak of famine disease had already occurred in spring 1941, but famine invaded the camps from August 1942 onwards.

> The first spell of cold weather led to a recrudescence of the disease, which spread rapidly throughout all the camps, creeping into every group, into all the huts, as though possessed of contagious characteristics. Though at first discreet, the symptoms became more and more evident, the trend more and more disquieting. In many ways the disease showed the classical signs observed during famines, but it also presented characteristics peculiar to the special environment of the camps throughout which it was spreading.[3]

The death rate continually increased revealing, after a period of resistance, the deep exhaustion and extreme physiological destitution of the weakened organisms of the inmates. Men appeared to be much less resistant than women, teenagers and children. Private relief organisations drew up a plan of action which found strong obstacles to its implementation, but was finally deployed with the help of large relief organisations and the goodwill of administrative authorities in the camps.

The plan comprised five main aspects: first of all, the examination of all internees from the point of view of their state of health and nutrition in order to spot inmates suffering from famine disease; hospitalisation of famine patients in special huts for observation and treatment; establishment of special dietetic kitchens under the joint responsibility of the relief organisations; emergency medical treatment consisting of dietetic products, vitamins, minerals and tonics, and segregation of threatened patients in a centre for prophylactic treatment separate from the camp. This medical relief intervention started in February 1942.

Internment camps became a big laboratory for clinical research on malnutrition and physical exhaustion under extreme circumstances. The medical program included screening all the inmates in order to select those patients showing nutritional deficiency syndrome. A clinical and therapeutic study of the sick hospitalised in the quarters for cachectic patients followed. The food situation was analysed, all activities of the relief organisations coordinated, doctors gave medical instructions to be followed and finally a critical examination of the results took place.

---

3 "Famine Disease," 1943-1944, p. 723.

In the course of a preliminary examination, all internees were weighed and measured, pulse-rate and blood pressure recorded as well as the main facts of their personal medical history. Patients were submitted to a simple medical examination in a subsequent examination and the results recorded on individual cards. A classification of the examined persons took place according to the following data: weight in relation to height; condition of the skin and subcutaneous tissue, muscular tone; station; cardiovascular system, oedema and blood counts. Patients were divided into three main categories: cachectic, pre-cachectic and threatened. Special infirmaries called cachectic quarters received those patients suffering from extreme skeleton-like emaciation. Many adults of medium height weighed only about 40 kilograms. Their physical condition was extremely impaired: dry skin, subicteric pallor, signs of cyanosis or haemolytic process, and anaemia. Pre-cachectic patients displayed the same symptoms but to a lesser degree, and their general condition was not so seriously damaged. Threatened cases were in better shape, with a tendency to show symptoms of hunger oedema, some emaciation and weakness. Most of these patients were convalescent from typhoid fever, gastric or duodenal ulcer, tuberculosis and chronic uncompensated cardiac disease. Based on the quantitative results for a camp with a population of about 11,000 internees of whom 9,000 were examined, 331 were classified as cachectic, 839 as pre-cachectic and about 4,000 were under the label of threatened cases.

"These proportions, however, were not static. *Famine disease*, which developed like a virulent epidemic, constantly progressed in the camps. Every week systematic investigation discovered new pre-cachectic and threatened cases, as though the virulence of the pathogenic agent were far from spent."[4] From the first results of the screening work, it appeared that more than half the inmates were threatened by symptoms of famine disease. This research on camp inmates allowed the definition of clinical forms of famine:

Humid famine: the principal form being hunger oedema.

Dry famine: characterised by the absence of oedema; it was most common among Spaniards and Italians, showing dry and scaly skin.

Anaemic famine: blood examination and neurological symptoms "of considerable pathogenic and therapeutic interest."

Circulatory famine: unstable blood pressure, hypotension, bradycardia showing heart suffering.

4 "Famine Disease," 1943-1944, p. 730.

Neurological famine: ataxia, paresthesia, polyneuritis symptoms, mixture of Parkinsonian and ataxic symptoms…

Mental famine: patients showed a "fixed, lifeless and apathetic gaze," confusion, prostration and extreme weakness.

The famine categories found in internment camps with their physical and physiological symptoms were carefully detailed in the published report.

> A more prolonged observation would certainly have permitted better classification of the various forms mentioned and the addition of some others. Nevertheless, the experience acquired during the investigations it was possible to make has clearly demonstrate the existence of these clinical forms in all the camps, one form or another preponderating according to the geographical situation of the centre and the origin of the internees.[5]

The determination of these clinical categories contributed to medical knowledge; they were also useful for prognosis and for the orientation of the treatment.

The genesis and evolution of the physical and mental impairment associated to the famine syndrome were followed carefully after the arrival of new internees in a normal state of nourishment. Those inmates were abruptly subjected to the camp fare. The deterioration of the general food supply and the growing destitution of the internees led to the appearance of the first symptoms of malnutrition at the end of 1942, "after a certain time-lag." A careful clinical observation of the internees revealed that once signs of nutritional deficiency appeared they followed each other in a particular order:

During the first three months of a deficient dietary, a heavy loss of weight took place, at a rhythm of 8 to 15 kilograms per month. After that initial period a gradually decreasing loss happened from month to month. A gradual disappearance of the fatty tissue was observed and inguinal hernia was frequent.

A general feeling of fatigue followed, accompanied by irritability and a change of the bodily complexion characterised by becoming straw-coloured, lemon-yellow, or white; dry skin, fugitive morning oedema, sometimes lasting for about ten minutes.

At a further stage headaches appeared, sometimes accompanied by mental disorders, depression or excitement, excited reflexes, static disturbances and amenorrhea in women. Finally, giddiness and ankle-cramps appeared, oedema became permanent, showing a tendency to

5 "Famine Disease," 1943-1944, p. 734-735.

generalisation and cardiac arrhythmia. At this point global impairment was so deep that if active intervention did not take place, the outcome of famine disease was inevitably death. Not only malnutrition was the cause; restrictions on freedom of movement, cold weather, unfavourable hygienic conditions, moral depression, that is to say the appalling living conditions could "only hasten this fatal development."[6]

The medical research program did not finish with the death of the patient; it included as well a careful and detailed observation of the conditions under which the death had happened, something considered by the medical experts "very instructive from the pathogenic point of view." The permanent impairment of physiological conditions finally led to a state of coma, followed, after a more or less short interval, by death. Sometimes, patients were suddenly struck down and collapsed while walking, sometimes they died in bed while sleeping.

Some patients passed away slowly, showing signs of progressive asthenia, or died from pre-existing or inter-current diseases. An autopsy was practiced, which usually revealed nothing macroscopically relevant, "apart from the occasional presence of cerebral oedema."[7]

The medical research programme was developed in two internment camps; mortality during January and February 1942 was

	January	February
Internment camp harbouring 400 people:	45	49
Internment camp harbouring 2,800 people:	59	38

Internment camps were endowed with technology to carry out clinical exploration: fluoroscopic examination, X-ray screening and blood analysis were applied to almost all the inmates. Cases of pulmonary tuberculosis were detected, as well as cardiovascular disturbances, such as heart enlargement and broncho-vascular infhammation.

> Angiospasm of the toes and finger-tips were often observed [...] but the condition cleared up with the administration of vitamins, and particularly nicotinic acid. Numerous cases of frost-bitten extremities were observed during winter, some of them very severe, necessitating, for instance, the amputation of fingers in two children. Many cases of *senile* opacity of the crystalline lens and frequent cases of precocious senility were also observed.[8]

6 "Famine Disease," 1943-1944, p. 735.

7 "Famine Disease," 1943-1944, p. 736.

8 "Famine Disease," 1943-1944, p. 737.

There was a striking decalcification of the bones, and osseous trabeculae were sometimes visible, such observations being typical of a deficiency condition. An abnormal degree of decalcification and demineralisation had taken place in the bones. Clinical and X-ray screening detected endocrine disorders. Hyperthyroid cases were rare but goitre was frequent; puberty was delayed in girls and a meaningful amount of women over fifteen and under 45 years suffered from amenorrhea. Adrenal alterations led to hypotension, hypoglycaemia and asthenia. Men suffered from alterations of spermatogenesis. Dysfunctions of genital endocrine glands suggested to the experts pituitary disturbances. On the contrary, diabetic patients seemed to benefit from deficient diet, as well as rheumatic, metabolic diseases.

Considered by medical researchers as an epidemic situation, the evolutionary curve showed, in a first phase, a progressive increase in morbidity, "consequent upon contamination, till it reaches a high level or a peak, and then falls again when a sufficiently large proportion of the population has acquired immunity, or when active measures effectively prevent the spread of the disease."[9] At the time when the medical research was brought to an end, famine disease had not reached its peak in the camps. Every week, the screening of the patients revealed new pre-cachectic and threatened cases, for the causes of the famine were far from having disappeared.

The gender divide showed important features. Women were affected after a time lag of ten months, as compared with men. Considering this fact, the increasing number of women affected by the deficiency syndrome in July 1942 was a clear expression of the general impairment of the general situation. Medical experts did not take into consideration external or social aspects, such as the intensity of physical work, which could contribute to explaining this situation. On the contrary, they stated that

> [...] the fact that the calorie requirements of women are 20% lower than those of man, and the slowing-up of metabolism due to amenorrhea, explain in part why they have been more resistant to famine than men. It appears that in the end their resistance broke down in its turn, and that the prognosis in the case of women became less favourable than it had previously been.[10]

On the other hand, climate conditions seemed to have a close influence upon evolution and survival. There was more chance of saving a patient during mild seasons than in wintertime. Cold climate had a weakening influence because calorie losses and existing vascular and

---

9 "Famine Disease," 1943-1944, p. 738.

10 "Famine Disease," 1943-1944, p. 739.

nervous disorders were aggravated. Patients who died in winter died as much from the cold as from famine. On the contrary, a warm temperature had positive effects over oedema. The medical report found that those patients suffering from neurological and mental forms of famine had the most negative prognosis, as well as the appearance of abundant diarrhoea, which is a cause of dehydration, demineralisation and bad assimilation of nutrients and vitamins.

Some signs indicated a fatal prognosis. The inability of patients to keep on their feet for some minutes showed a serious situation. Medical experts found indispensable prescribing strict and complete rest if those patients were to be protected from sudden death. Also, pronounced atrophy and extreme emaciation accompanied cachexia, and, a as a general rule, patients already suffering from other diseases got worse due to famine.

The medical research experts responded to famine disease as if it were not a social problem provoked by living conditions at the internment camps but a sort of epidemic affordable from a purely medical and scientific perspective. The possibilities of cure they considered depended upon age, season, early institution of treatment and the extent of the therapeutic action undertaken. They were explicit: "[...] an incurable condition (apart from terminal coma) does not exist. Notwithstanding a remarkable loss of weight, profound asthenia and a very serious general condition, it was found possible, through *persevering an energetic treatment*, to save individuals considered to be irrevocably lost."[11] Treatment being based on a substantial diet rich in fats and proteins, and on hypertonic injections of glucose, the medical research found that patients were saved who had been considered hopeless cases, suffering from generalised oedema, ascites, pleural effusion, myocarditis, hemorrhagic purpura and losing as much as 55% of their physiological weight. Segregation of severe cases was considered to be an indispensable therapeutic factor, especially for those suffering from mental disorders.

One of the experimental targets of the research project was to assess the exact role played by vitamin deficiency in famine disease. However, the exact participation of it in clinical signs and physical deterioration was impossible to ascertain. Obviously, experts easily discovered the consequences of a deficient calorie intake, such as emaciation, loss of weight and disappearance of fat, but clinical examination did not enable them to assess specific signs resulting from the lack of any definite vitamin. "Moreover, the vitamin requirements of the human body can vary and be subject at the same time to individual factors and to en-

11 "Famine Disease," 1943-1944, p. 740.

dogenous influences, which govern the absorption and utilisation of the vitamins consumed."[12] They talked about clinical symptoms related to vitamin C, D, A, vitamins, nicotinamide and decalcification.

Indeed, the medical report found obvious that the miserable physical condition of the internees was due to the inadequacy of their diet, both from the quantity and quality of food. A simple comparison between the indispensable elements of a normal diet and the one served to the inmates of the camps offered an evident conclusion.

Famine disease was considered the consequence of a chronic quantitative and qualitative deficiency in the diet. The daily rations, expressed in calories, provided in a camp during one month from October 1st to 30th, 1942 per person was as follows:

Foodstuff	Grams	Calories
Bread	7,500	17,000
Fats	240	2,160
Sugar	480	1,960
Pumpkin[a]	30,000	6,100
Jam	2,250	2,250
Sardines	1,800	1,674
Cheese	200	600
Meat	913	911
Tripe	770	465
Carrots	3,750	1,406
Cabbage[b]	3,750	1,125

[a] morning and evening for three weeks
[b] carrots and cabbage morning and evening for a week

The calorie intake calculated was 1,188 calories per person per day (35,651:30) resulting from an average daily intake of:

Proteins (animal origin)	15
Proteins (vegetal origin)	37
Fats (animal origin)	12
Fats (vegetal origin)	2
Carbohydrates	210

It was accepted that about 15% to 20% of the theoretical energy value of nutrients in diet was in reality lost, therefore the actual value of the daily ration per person was not 1,188 calories, but around 950

[12] "Famine Disease," 1943-1944, p. 741.

calories a day on average. As we analysed in previous chapters, in 1942, a great deal of experimental and clinical research on nutrition had established solid patterns regarding calorie intake necessities for health. A lot of technical reports and articles were available about the consequences of shortage and malnutrition during the Great War, from 1914 to 1918. The situation was considered to be critical when daily protein intake fell to 40-50 grams per day, fats intake to 20-30 grams, and daily calorie value between 1,400 and 1,800.

The daily protein ration in the internment camps was not more than 30 to 40 grams of almost exclusively vegetal origin and fats intake was 8 to 10 grams a day, which in no case allowed protein balance to be maintained. When the protein ration and the calorie intake fall simultaneously below the physiological minimum, not only nitrogen balance is upset, but also the elimination of proteins gets abnormally increased. Cachexia cannot be overcome even by giving large amounts of fats and carbohydrates, and weight cannot increase if the minimum requirement of proteins is not supplied. Instead of one gram of protein per kilo of body weight defined as necessary by nutritionists, the diet provided only 48 grams of vegetal protein. A continual nitrogen deficit followed, which, even though it amounted to only 9 grams a day, represented for these internees 3,300 grams of protein in the course of a year, a serious impairment of the muscles and other organs being the consequence. The same vegetables were served for weeks on end. Besides, they were badly prepared, inadequately stored and for too long. A meaningful amount of inmates suffered from intestinal disorders, and defective absorption was yet another factor of vitamin deficiency even though the intake was adequate.

Medical researchers then made a comparison with the food situation of a large industrial town near the camps, in collaboration with the Nutrition Section of the Regional Hygiene Institute. Quantitative data for February 1941 showed that the average for different social groups was 1,737 calories for adults and 1,565 calories for teenagers. The lowest figures accepted by physiologists were 1,600 calories for male adults, 1,400 for female adults and 1,400 for teenagers. At the end of 1941 figures were similar: for the least favoured group, 1,764 calories per male adult, 1,509 per female adult and 1,614 per teenager.

Based on these figures, the experts compared the food situation in the town to that of German towns in 1917. As to the food situation in the camps, the ration average was not unlike that in Madrid towards the end of the siege, during the civil war, when the ration was 852 calories (it was 1,514 calories at the beginning of the siege).[13] From the comparative study, medical experts concluded that the ration supplied to the internees in the camps was 40% to 50% lower than that of the civilian population of the nearby industrial town, which was itself seriously affected by a food shortage. They predicted that the *epidemic of famine disease* would persist in the camps and that the efforts of the organisations to combat the situation by supplying additional nourishment and intensive drug therapy would remain ineffective under the existing conditions. It was urgent to raise the ration in all the camps to the level of the civil population.

> If the efforts made by the organisations on behalf of the cachectic patients in the special quarters provided for them had been supported by a similar effort on behalf of the inmates of the entire camps, it might really have been possible to save them all. For this, it would have sufficed to make sure that the internees were receiving the strict ration to which they were entitled.[14]

Relief organisations made considerable efforts sending supplementary foodstuffs to the camps but, according to the medical report, failure was due to the insufficient food rations given to the internees. When the relief organisations discovered that famine disease was spreading in the internment camps, they intensified their efforts; several kitchens were installed especially designed to feed cachectic patients, who received a daily ration from 2,200 to 2,500 calories, with an appreciable improvement of the quality. Relief organisations sought to procure a nourishing diet, scientifically calculated and adapted to patients in a state of advanced cachexia. On the other hand, to stop the *famine epidemic*, they supplied an ever-growing number of *threatened* patients with food supplements in the form of pea or rice soups, pasta, pearl barley or dried or fresh fruit, accounting for some 250 to 400 calories.

> It is impossible in the present study to give an adequate idea of the immense effort exerted by the organisations engaged in relief work, the flexibility of their action and the spirit of co-operation animating them. Some inkling of it may be given by the fact that in less than a week the kitchens were installed; that a detailed card-index was prepared and kept up-to-date containing the follow-up observations concerning patients cared for by each organisation; that most of the necessary foodstuffs were purchased in the Balkans, Turkey, Portugal and Spain, and that others were despatched from the two Americas; that storehouses were built; and a great deal of work done in connection with the handling and storing of the supplies. When we add that, in addition to these material arrangements, many necessary negotiations were undertaken with the authorities on behalf of the internees either in general or

---

13 "Famine Disease," 1943-1944, p. 750; Grande Covián, 1939, p. 22.

14 "Famine Disease," 1943-1944, p. 752.

in individual cases, a fair idea is given of the impressive work carried out jointly on behalf of the internees by a dozen international and national relief organisations.[15]

The work of the organisations covered from 65% to 70% of the internees in the camp. In June 1942, 1,958 rations a day were distributed among 2,750 inmates in one large camp. Specific action took place in the maternity section, where the weight of the newly-born infants shifted from an average of 2.1 kilograms to 2.5 kilograms in 1941 to 2.9 kilograms to 3.1 kilograms in 1942 and 1943. No infant mortality rates appeared in the medical report.

Some sort of drug therapy was also implemented depending on the various clinical forms of famine. Patients suffering from *dry famine* were supplemented with tonics, drugs containing amino-acids, stimulants, vitamins and phosphorus-containing products. In those affected by *humid famine*, diuretics were added to the above and, for patients affected by *neurological and mental famine*, brewers' yeast, glucose and aneurin were added. In cases of anaemia, iron extracts and vitamins were administered. The effects of a wide range of drugs was evaluated: brewers' yeast, calcium, glucose, iron, insulin, coramin, vitamin A, B, C, D and E, nicotinamide, hepatogastric extract, wheat germ, ortedrin, pervitin, sulphonamides. All this medical treatment was accompanied by rest and segregation for constant care and by systematic supervision in the case of cachectic and pre-cachectic patients.

According to the evaluation of the medical experts, dietary and drug treatment had completely changed the appearance and condition of the patients. The decline in mortality followed an abrupt tendency, once relief had been well organised. During the last two weeks of April 1942, in 100 cachectic patients from a camp, an increase in weight was recorded in 32%, a stationary condition in 20%, a loss of weight owing to a decrease in fluid (oedema) in 40%, and a real loss of weight in 8% of the cases. During the first half of May, the number of cachectic patients who gained weight reached 60.4%. But after the medical programme of intervention and the two months of therapeutic experience, the cachectic and pre-cachectic patients who returned to everyday life at the camp relapsed because they were still exposed to the same pathogenic factor: famine.

> The inadequacy and the irregularities of the rations effectively supplied to the inmates by the administrative authorities of the camps made it impossible definitely to save them. Those who were saved from the consequences of famine at the cost of great effort on the part of the relief organisations in

---

[15] "Famine Disease," 1943-1944, p. 753.

> supplying supplements of food would thus be still suspended sentence of death, unless the camp authorities supplied them with a more or less adequate basic ration, this basic ratio remaining the prime factor in the problem of saving famine-disease patients. When all is said and done, the obligation to solve this problem rested with the authorities responsible for the internment of the inmates of the camps.[16]

At the end of the medical report, a postscript was added:

> The changes in the military and political situation in Europe which have taken place since this study was written and set up enable us now to lift the veil of anonymity from its authors, from the organisations to which they belong, from the scene of their labours and from the bodies which supplied them with the wherewithal to carry out their work.
>
> The study is, to a great extent, based on a report dated July 1942 of the "health Commission" of the "Co-ordination Committee for Relief in Camps," consisting of Dr. Rene Zimmer, representing the Unitarian Service Committee of the United States, Dr. Maurice Dubois, of the Swiss Red Cross, Children's Relief (*Secours aux Infants*) and Dr. Joseph Weill, of the O.S.E. Union (Jewish health organisation).
>
> Dr Weill was obliged very considerably to modify the text of the original report in order to enable it to be published and to incorporate later information in it.
>
> The camps in which the observations were recorded are situated in the south of France and, more particularly, in the Eastern Pyrenees. They were organised in 1939 and 1940, in the first place to accommodate Spanish refugees, whence their name of *Centres d'hébergement*, and then, during the first part of the world war, to receive "enemy aliens."

From July 1940, these camps were mainly filled with Jews of various nationalities. During the second half of 1942, tens of thousands of them were deported from the camps of Poland.

The camps designated by the letters "G..." and "R..." are those at Gurs and Rivesaltes respectively. The town, the food rations of which, have been indicated for purposes of comparison with those of camps in Marseille.

The charitable organisations which took part in the provision of relief for the internees were the following:

Aide aux Émigrés, Swiss section of the International Migration Service, Geneva;

The Confederation of Swiss Jewish Communities

The Joint relief Committee of the International Red Cross;

---

16 "Famine Disease," 1943-1944, p. 761.

The Ecumenical Council, Geneva;

O.S.E. Union (Jewish Health organisation), Geneva;

Schweizerischer Aerzte verein (Swiss medical union), Zurich;

Secours Suisse aux enfants, Geneva;

The Society of Friends, United States;

The Swiss Red Cross;

The Unitarian Service Committee, United States.

Furthermore, consignments of medicaments were supplied free of cost by the following manufacturers of pharmaceutical products in Basle: C. Boehringer & Co., C.I.B.A., Geigy, and Sandoz, to whom the authors desire to express their gratitude...[17]

[17] "Famine Disease," 1943-1944, p. 772.

Conclusion

The great international crisis experienced by Europe between 1914 and 1945 gave political, economic and social priority to food availability and the problems of hunger and diet. As a consequence of the crisis caused by the First World War, international conflicts and the 1929 stock market crash, food production and consumption became a State responsibility and the role of experimental science not only influenced knowledge, but also inspired agricultural and health policies, and had effects on the economy, education and cultural habits. The *problem of nutrition* took on a plural dimension, becoming central in wartime and after a war. In this particular context, international experts became principal agents for the development of public health and social welfare policies. Hunger and poverty became an economic and political problem, and a problem pertaining to health.

Consequently, international organisations, in collaboration with states and philanthropic associations, pushed experimental research and launched field studies on the diet, as well as campaigns to coordinate food production with trade demands, according to the principles of the new science of nutrition. The League of Nations, the International Labour Office, the International Institute of Agriculture, the Rockefeller Foundation, all them became major agents. During the interwar period, diet and nutrition became an excellent argument to explore the relationships between the genesis of scientific knowledge, political and commercial uses, and social and political practices. Researching the plural factors involved, allowed us to analyse the mechanisms behind the origin and transfer of scientific knowledge.

The great convulsion experienced by European societies during the three decades from 1914 to 1945 prompted the State as an element of social stabilisation in national and international conflicts, and accentuated its regulatory role on the economy and citizens' health. The policies on diet and nutrition implemented between 1920 and 1945 were a great failure from the point of view of production, trade and health, one that was utterly dramatic to human health, with situations of famine spreading in large regions of Europe since the beginning of the Spanish Civil War until the post-war years of the Second World War. However, that exceptional situation turned the whole of Europe into a vast laboratory for the development of the science of nutrition, for the study of the effects of nutritional deficiencies on human health, for the massive clinical exploration of the population, and for the development of an industry around food and deficiency disease. Laboratory research, industry and market made food and nutrition a central clue for social development.

Indeed, during the interwar years the physiology of nutrition received a strong stimulus due to a social interest in evaluating the impact of the international crisis on health. A balanced diet came to be considered essential for the establishment of the optimum health needed to fight off infectious diseases. It was considered to be the basis of organic energy. On the contrary, mere *consumption* was considered to be the negative consequence of deficient nutrition, an early stage of infection and organic impairment. School canteens and meals for workers, mothers and poor people constituted a field where social policies had a clear international dimension. The close interaction between the international context and national politics was evident in the case of agricultural policies, food production, food availability and experimental research on nutrition and diet. The League of Nations played a coordinating role by means of a Technical Commission on Nutrition that developed not only experimental research but also clinical and somatometric tests to identify deficiency diseases and prevent malnutrition. An international group of experts worked together establishing a powerful reference for nutritional politics and health standards. Its constitution was promoted by the LoN together with the International Labour Office and the International Institute of Agriculture. Expert committees and international conferences encouraged experimental research to ascertain optimum standards for each country; they tried to ensure that medical students, medical officers and district nurses, teachers and civil servants received the latest nutritional knowledge, and encouraged a vigorous policy of education for the general public.

Pregnant women, infants and children, peasants and workers became the main target of an internationally connected policy including laboratory research, clinical screening, dietary standards for low incomes and previously defined social groups at risk (rural areas, children, pregnant women, peasants, industrial workers, the unemployed, etc.). Food and diet were not only a matter of economy, physiology and survival; new trends in community nutrition became a political tool to overcome a critical period and civilise people according to scientific patterns and liberal values. Technical reports discussed dietary standards, especially concerning infants and families with small incomes, criteria for an optimum diet, the nutritive value of foodstuffs as well as methods of screening the nutritional state of the population.

Technical reports by experts in nutrition achieved legitimacy in the eyes of politicians as a reference for food production and as a way to instruct popular habits at a time in which the food industry gained momentum. National policies received legitimation from international experts on nutrition science and community initiatives were reinforced by the international context. As a consequence, the new science of nutrition became a political tool and one of the main loci of action in the big programme of civilisation developed in Western countries during the first half of the 20th century. It was a field of knowledge and action to overcome famine, malnutrition, deficiencies in the production of foodstuffs and change habits according to new bourgeois, liberal values.

Nevertheless, the crises represented by the Spanish Civil War and the Second World War changed the international panorama and the high hopes attached to the science of nutrition, as the nucleus of social change collapsed. A general deterioration of the living conditions occurred, and food availability became a central concern in most countries. In fact, food became a military tool influencing the development of the war in many places. Thus, in the 1940s deficiency illnesses were identified and evaluated by a technically and conceptually solid science of nutrition that was, however, unable to alleviate the underlying hunger. Internment camps were the most dramatic laboratory of research for extreme, seriously impaired situation. Experimental and clinical screening of inmates in internment camps, being an argument for health and charitable intervention, exceeded all limits of respect to human dignity and civil rights. The intervention of experimental science to analyse, identify and classify famine and a variety of malnutrition and nutrition deficiencies in internment camps was a sort of tragic comedy in which doctors faced the problem as an epidemic problem. The new science of nutrition was useful in identifying the problems, in building experimental knowledge on the wrecker effects of famine, its sequence and limits, but was impotent in offering practical solutions.

The international situation changed later during the Cold War, although international agencies continued to play a positive but limited role. Initially, the Food and Agriculture Organisation (FAO) turned out to be a more conservative body than many internationalists had hoped, focusing on improved living conditions rather than on eliminating world hunger. Proposals for a world food board by the first director general of the FAO, Boyd Orr, were sidelined."[1]

The new approach to a global food policy went hand in hand with the development of what more recently has been called global civil society,

1 Staples 2006, p. 32.

a less developed face of globalisation. The significance of cooperatives for mutual aid and democratic culture as well as for agricultural production and distribution had been stressed by the FAO since its birth at the Hot Springs conference in May 1943.[2] Yet, today's global market, based on exploitation and not on equity, still lacks the instruments and capacity of regulation needed to fight global hunger. The incapacity of capitalism as a global system and the limited influence of international and national, public and private initiatives to challenge the problem of food availability and nutrition by means of a wise combination of science, production, market and politics have delayed the unsolved problem until the present days.

2 Staples 2006, p. 38.

References

Documents and Technical Reports

The documents and technical reports listed below belong to the Historical Archives of the League of Nations (Geneva) and the FAO Archives (Rome).

Historical Archives of the League of Nations, Geneva

1926, *Nutrition*, R.990.

1928-1935, *Nutrition: general*, R.5865-5866.

1929, *Food Supplies: reparation and distribution*, R.5910.

1929-1932, *Food Supplies: Preparations alleged to contain vitamins*, R.5910.

1930-1932, *Food Supplies: Standardisation of vitamins*, R.5921 and R.6078-79.

1932, *Food Supplies: Distribution of vitamin standards*, R.5935 and R.6009.

1932-1933, *Étude de l'état alimentaire*, R.5936.

1932-1933, *Études sur la meilleure utilisation, pour l'alimentation des budgets réduits*, R.5936.

Introductory note on the work accomplished (History and method) by the League of Nations up to October 1935 (Nutrition), 1935, 12 p. [C.H.1194].

League of Nations Health Organisation. Technical Commission on Nutrition, *On the Food Problem of the Civil Population of Madrid*, August 1938. [C.H./Com.Exp.Alim./57] R.6135/8A/23831/20883.

League of Nations Health Organisation. Technical Commission on Nutrition, "Report by a Special Committee which met in Geneva... 1938," *League of Nations Bulletin of the Health Organisation*, 7, (1938), p. 666-678. [C.H.1355, 10p.M.].

Memorandum on nutrition and health, prepared by the Health Section for the Mixed Committee on the problem of Nutrition, 1936, 30 p. [C.H.1204].

Milk and Milk Products in Sweden (Studies on nutrition), 1926. [C.H./Com.Exp.Alim./5: Divers/I].

[Note on] the Conference on Rural Life and the Problem of Nutrition, 1938, 4 p. [C.H./Com.Exp.Alim./44].

Problem of nutrition with special reference to rural districts, Geneva, 1935, 4 p. [C.H./Hyg.rur./E.H./3].

Relation of Nutrition to Health, Agriculture and Economy Policy. Final report of the mixed Committee of the League of Nations, Geneva, 1937, 340 p. [A.13.1937, 1937.II.A.10].

Report on the Physiological Basis of Nutrition drawn up by the Technical Commission of the Health Committee at the meeting held in London (November 25th-29th, 1935) [C.H.1197], revised and amplified at the meeting held at Geneva (June 4th-8th, 1936), Geneva, 1936. [A.12(1).1936.II.B].

Report of the Sub-Committee on Nutrition (Meeting of the Directors of National Schools and Institutes of Hygiene in Europe), Geneva, 1937, 6 p. [C.H.1298].

Report on the health situation in Spain, Rockefeller Foundation, 20 August 1939. Rockefeller Archive Centre, New York, 1939.

Saiki, T., *Progress of the Science of Nutrition in Japan*, Geneva, 1926. [C.H.523].

Saiki, T., *Necessity of the study of nutrition*, Geneva, [1927], 8 p. [Doc. C.H.558].

Statistics of food production, consumption and prices. Documentation prepared by the International Institute of Agriculture, presented to the Mixed Committee on the Problem of Nutrition at its second session, June 4th, 1936. [A.12(c).1936.II.B].

Stiebeling, H.K., *The State of the L.O.N. in investigations of problems of food and nutrition*, Geneva, [1938], 21 p. [C.H./Com.Exp.Alim/51].

Technical Commission on Nutrition. Documentation, League of Nations health Organisation. 3rd session, London, 15th November 1937. [R.6134, 8a, 23831, 20883: Docs: C.H./Com.Exp.Alim/33, C.H./Com.Exp.Alim/26, C.H./Com.Exp.Alim/27, C.H./Com.Exp.Alim/28, C.H./Com.Exp.Alim/12, C.H./Com.Exp.Alim/13, C.H./Com.Exp.Alim/15, C.H./Com.Exp.Alim/16, C.H./Com.Exp.Alim/18, C.H./Com.Exp.Alim/19, C.H./Com.Exp.Alim/30, C.H./Com.Exp.Alim/32, C.H./Com.Exp.Alim/35, C.H. 1261, C.H., 1216]

Tsurumi, M., *Notes communiquées par le Dr... à la 22e session du Comité Hygiène (7-16.10.1935). Sur l'alimentation*, 6 p. [C.H. 1173].

FAO Archives, Rome

Données sur la FAO, Organisation des Nations Unies pour l'Agriculture et l'Alimentation, Washington, 1947. [BGE Zt 2598/12].

Enquête Mondiale sur l'Alimentation, Washington, Rome, Organisation des Nations Unies pour l'Agriculture et l'Alimentation, 1946-1953. [Cote QU 146.1 53OR HIST].

Joint FAO/WHO Espert Committee on Nutrition. Report on the first session, Geneva, World Health Organisation, 1950.

Joint FAO/WHO Espert Committee on Nutrition. Prevention and treatment of severe malnutrition in times of disaster. Presented to World Health Assembly, Geneva, World Health Organisation, 1951.

Joint FAO/WHO Espert Committee on Nutrition, Rome April 10th-17th 1951. Past activities and future program.

Rapport de la Réunion de la FAO sur la Nutrition en Europe, Rome, Food and Agriculture Organisation, 1958, 28 p. [QU 146. GA1 58OR HIST].

World Food Survey [1st], Washington, Food and Agriculture Organisation, 1946, 39 p. [QU 146.1 46FO HIST].

World Food Survey [2nd], Rome, Food and Agriculture Organisation, 1952, 59 p. [QU 146.1 52FO HIST].

Printed Sources

Aldecoa y Juarista, J.L., "Contribución al estudio de la lactancia materna (experiencias de guerra en Bilbao)," *Revista de Sanidad e Higiene Pública*, 1938/1939, Vol. 1, p. 241-245.

Alvarado, C., Pastor, M. A., "Estudio de la composición química de algunos alimentos españoles," *Revista de Sanidad e Higiene Pública*, 1933, Vol. 8, No. 4, p. 366-370.

Anguera A., "Servicios sanitarios con motivo de la inmigración durante la guerra," *Revista de Sanidad e Higiene Pública*, 1938/1939, Vol. 1, p. 25-42.

Annual report of the Chief Medical Officer of the Ministry of Health for the year 1933, League of Nations, Geneva, 1934.

Arias Vallejo, E., "Dietas fisiológicas, máxima y mínima en el régimen de alimentación del hombre adulto," *Revista de Sanidad e Higiene Pública*, 1943, p. 290-304.

Arias Vallejo, E., *Alimentación y síndromes carenciales*, Ediciones Morata, Madrid, 1943.

Aykroyd, W.R., "Diet in relation to small incomes," *League of Nations Quarterly Bulletin of the Health Organisation*, 1933, Vol. 1, p. 130-153.

Aykroyd, W.R., "The poor rice-eater's diet," *League of Nations Bulletin of the Health organisation*, 1940, Vol. 10, p. 342-356.

"Bibliography of the Technical Work of the Health Organisation of the League of Nations, 1920-1945," *League of Nations Bulletin of the Health Organisation*, 1945, Vol. 11.

Bigwood, E.J., Roost, G., *L'alimentation rationnelle et les besoins énergétiques d'une population ouvrière*, Université Libre de Bruxelles, Institut Solvay, Bruxelles, 1934.

Bigwood, E.J., *Guiding Principles for Studies On the Nutrition of Populations. Technical Commission on Nutrition*, Health Organisation of the League of Nations, Geneva, 1939. [C.H.1401; C.H./Com.Exp.Alim./50(2)].

Biraud, M., "Health in Europe. A Survey of the Epidemic and Nutritional Situation," *League of Nations Bulletin of the Health Organisation*, 1943-1944, Vol. 10, p. 557-699.

Blankenstein H. van, *L'Organisation d'Hygiène de la Société des Nations*, J. Musses, Purmerend, 1934.

Bootello, A., "Nuestros primeros resultados en la determinación del yodo en los alimentos y aguas de España," in *Contribución al I Congreso Nacional de Sanidad del laboratorio de Higiene de la Alimentación y de la Nutrición y Técnica Bromatológica*, Escuela Nacional de Sanidad, Madrid, 1934, p. 87-94.

Bourne, G.H., *Starvation in Europe*, Allen & Unwin, London, 1943.

Burnet, E., Aykroyd, W.R., 'Nutrition and Public Health," *League of Nations Quarterly Bulletin of the Health Organisation*, 1935, Vol. 4, No. 2, p. 323-474.

Calderón, A.M., "Vitaminas y sordera. Experiencia carencial del Madrid rojo: julio de 1936-marzo de 1939," *Revista de Sanidad e Higiene Pública*, 1940, Vol. 2, p. 420-445.

Calleja, C., *Guía para individualizar el régimen alimenticio con especial referencia a la edad y a la crasis o constitución*, Administración de la Revista de Medicina y Cirugía Prácticas, Madrid, 1911.

Carrasco Cadenas, E., *Ni gordos, ni flacos. Lo que se debe comer*, Diana, Madrid, 1935.

Carrasco Cadenas, E., "Escuela Nacional de Sanidad. Sección de Higiene de la Alimentación y de la Nutrición y Técnica Bromatológica. Su orientación y programa de trabajo al año y medio de su organización," *Revista de Sanidad e Higiene Pública*, 1933, Vol. 8, p. 258-260.

Carrasco Cadenas, E., "Lo que se come en España. Interés sanitario de este problema," in *Contribución al I Congreso Nacional de Sanidad del laboratorio de Higiene de la Alimentación y de la Nutrición y Técnica Bromatológica*, Escuela Nacional de Sanidad, Madrid, 1934a, p. 5-24.

Carrasco Cadenas, E., "Lo que se come en España. Interés sanitario de este problema," *Archivos de Medicina, Cirugía y Especialidades*, 1934b, Vol. 37, No. 25, p. 669-675.

Carrasco Cadenas, E., "Alteraciones oculares, dentarias, de crecimiento y desarrollo general en relación con el insuficiente aporte proteínico, de minerales y vitaminas, *Progresos de la Clínica*, 1934c, Vol. 42, p. 563-571.

Carrasco Cadenas, E., "Datos para suponer una carencia general vitamínica en algunas regiones españolas," in *Contribución al I Congreso Nacional de Sanidad del laboratorio de Higiene de la Alimentación y de la Nutrición y Técnica Bromatológica*, Escuela Nacional de Sanidad, Madrid, 1934d, p. 95-104.

Carrasco Cadenas, E., "Datos para suponer una carencia general vitamínica en algunas regiones españolas," *Archivos de Medicina, Cirugía y Especialidades*, 1934e, Vol. 37, No. 19, p. 501-503.

Carrasco Cadenas, E., *Sobre las necesidades alimenticias de la mujer. El problema de las vitaminas en la alimentación doméstica*, Aguilar, Madrid, 1934f.

Carrasco Cadenas, E., *Temas de higiene alimenticia de urgente atención sanitaria*, Escuela Nacional de Sanidad, Madrid, 1934g.

Carrasco Cadenas, E., Piñoles, L., "La riqueza vitamínica de algunos alimentos españoles. Primeros resultados obtenidos para el tomate valenciano y aceite de oliva andaluz," *Revista de Sanidad e Higiene Pública*, 1933, Vol. 8, No. 1, p. 1-22.

Carrasco Cadenas, E., Jiménez, F., Bootello, A., Alvarado, C., "La eliminación de yodo por la orina en los individuos normales sometidos a la sal yodada," in *Contribución al I Congreso Nacional de Sanidad del laboratorio de Higiene de la Alimentación y de la Nutrición y Técnica Bromatológica*, Escuela Nacional de Sanidad, Madrid, 1934, p. 75-86.

Carrasco Cadenas, E., Olmeda, C., "Contribución al estudio de la riqueza vitamínica de los alimentos españoles," in *Contribución al I Congreso Nacional de Sanidad del laboratorio de Higiene de la Alimentación y de la Nutrición y Técnica Bromatológica*, Escuela Nacional de Sanidad, Madrid, 1934, p. 105-133.

Chodzko W., *The Rural Centre for Public Health and Social Welfare and the Improvement of Rural Health Conditions, Sixteenth Session of the Health Committee*, League of Nations, Geneva, 1930.

Comenge, M., *Análisis de Alimentos*, Anastasio Medina, Toledo, 1934.

Comenge, M., *Principios bioquímicos de Dietética Normal y Tabla de composición de los alimentos españoles*, Madrid, 1948, 206 p.

"Conference of Experts for the Standardisation of Certain Methods used in making Dietary Studies. Held in Rome on September 2nd and 3rd, 1932," *League of Nations Quarterly Bulletin of the Health Organisation*, 1932, Vol. 1, No. 1, p. 477-483.

Conferencias sobre alimentación. Publicaciones de la Comisaría General de Abastecimientos y Transportes, Madrid, 1944, 199 p.

Cosin, J., *Estado actual de los standard internacionales de hormonas y vitaminas*, Imprenta de J. Cosano, Madrid, 1941.

Coward, K.H., "The relative antirachitic potencies of vitamin D2 (calciferol from irradiated ergosterol) and of vitamin D3 (from irradiated 7-dehydrocholesterol). A summary of experiments organised for the Accesory Food Factors Committee. (Lister Institute and Medical Research Council), *League of Nations Bulletin of the Health organisation*, 1940/41, Vol. 9, p. 425-435.

"Cuadro de las vitaminas y distribución de las más importantes. Instituto Nacional de Higiene de la Alimentación," *La voz de la Sanidad*, 1938, Vol. 1, 5 p.

"Current Notes on the Work of the Health Organisation. Conference on Nutrition," *League of Nations Quarterly Bulletin of the Health Organisation*, 1932, Vol. 1, No. 1, p. 311.

Dantín Cereceda J., *La alimentación española. Sus diferentes tipos*, Introducción, edición e índice onomástico de Juan Riera. Acta Histórico-Médica Vallisoletana, Valladolid, 1934.

"Economic Depression and Public Health, Memorandum prepared by the Health Section. III. The Nutrition of the Unemployed," *League of Nations Quarterly Bulletin of the Health Organisation*, 1932, Vol. 1, p. 443-457.

"Famine Disease and its Treatment in Internment Camps," *League of Nations Bulletin of the Health Organisation*, 1943-1944, Vol. 10, p. 722-772.

FAO, *Standing advisory comité on nutrition. First report to the director-general. Nutrition Division*, Copenhague 23-31 August, 1946, FAO, Washington, 1946.

FAO, *Report of the special meeting on urgent food problems*, FAO, Washington, 1946.

FAO, *World Food Survey. Monograph living worldwide nutrition statistics and food production statistics by continent and country. Figures and proteins from pre-war food supplies and nutritional targets in several areas, pre-war food consumption survey, food production statistics per head of population*, FAO, Rome, 1946.

FAO, *The Nutritive Value of Foods. Conference*, FAO, Montevideo, 1948.

FAO, *Note on Nutrition and Agriculture. Nutrition Conference*, FAO, Montevideo, 1948.

FAO, *Food composition tables. Nutrition Division*, FAO, Washington, 1948.

FAO, *Nutrition education. Third Meeting of the Standing Advisory Committee on Nutrition*, FAO, Washington, 1948.

FAO, *Food composition tables of international use*, FAO, Washington, 1949.

FAO/WHO, *Joint FAO/WHO expert committee on nutrition*, FAO/WHO, Geneva, 1949.

Final Report of the Mixed Committee of the League of Nations on Relation of Nutrition to Health, Agriculture and Economic Policy, League of Nations, Geneva, 1937. [A.13.1937.II.A].

Food and the War, United States Food Administration, Boston, 1918.

García Luquero, "Aspectos sanitarios de la evacuación de refugiados en Santander," *Revista de Sanidad e Higiene Pública*, 1938-1939, Vol. 1, p. 68-81.

García Triviño F., "Predisposición y tuberculosis," *Revista de Higiene y Tuberculosis*, 1914, Vol. 8, p. 4-6.

Giral, J., *Ración alimenticia desde los puntos de vista higiénico y social*, Adrián Romo Editor, Madrid, 1914.

Giral, J., "Repercusiones económicas y sociales de la alimentación humana. Conferencia dada en la Escuela Nacional de Sanidad el 24 de mayo de 1934," *Revista de Sanidad e Higiene Pública*, 1934, p. 121-139.

Godoy Ramírez, J., *Vitaminas y avitaminosis*, Sempere, Almería, 1922.

Gómez Ocaña, J., *Los alimentos minerales. Discurso leído en la solemne sesión inaugural del año de 1914 ... en la Real Academia de Medicina.* Real Academia Nacional de Medicina, Madrid, 1914.

González Campo, J., *La alimentación de las clases pobres de Madrid como factor etiológico de enfermedades gástricas e intestinales*, Idamor Moreno, Madrid, 1903.

Gorter, E., De Lange, C., "Nutritive food requirements during the first year of life," *League of Nations Bulletin of the Health Organisation*, 1937, Vol. 6, No. 2, p. 291-298.

Grande Covián, F., *La alimentación en Madrid durante la Guerra. (Estudio de la dieta suministrada a la población civil madrileña durante diecinueve meses de guerra: Agosto 1937 a Febrero 1939)*, Publicación de la Revista de Sanidad e Higiene Pública, 1939.

Grande Covián, F., Jiménez García, F., "Sobre los trastornos carenciales observados en Madrid durante la Guerra. II. Presentación en el tiempo de los distintos cuadros carenciales," *Revista Clínica Española*, 1940, Vol. 1, p. 318-322.

Grande Covián, F., Jiménez García, F., "Algunas observaciones acerca de la acción del ácido nicotínico sobre la glucemia y la lactacidemia," *Revista Clínica Española*, 1940, Vol. 1, p. 325-329.

Grande Covián, F., Jiménez García, F., "El contenido en ácido nicotínico de las dietas consumidas en Madrid durante la guerra," *Revista Clínica Española*, 1943, Vol. 8, p. 28-30.

Grande Covián, F., Jiménez García, F., "El tratamiento de la pelagra por el ácido nicotínico," *Revista Clínica Española*, 1940, Vol. 1, p. 49-81.

Grande Covián, F., "Sobre el peso de los recién nacidos, durante la guerra en Madrid," *Revista Clínica Española*, 1940, Vol. 1, p. 501-504.

Grande Covián, F., "La secreción láctea durante la hipoalimentación. (observaciones en las madres lactantes de Madrid durante la guerra)," *Revista Clínica Española*, 1940, Vol. 1, p. 180-188.

Grande Covián, F., "Dietas fisiológicas, máxima y mínima en el régimen de alimentación del hombre adulto," *Revista de Sanidad e Higiene Pública*, 1943, p. 115-129.

Grande Covián, F., "L'alimentation et les troubles alimentaires durant la Guerre Civile Espagnole," in *Les Vitaminas*, Bâle, Roche, 1944.

Grande Covián, F., Peraita, M., *Avitaminosis y Sistema Nervioso*, Miguel Server, Barcelona, 1941a.

Grande Covián, F., *La ciencia de la alimentación*, Ediciones Pegaso, Madrid, 1947.

Grande Covián, F., Peraita, M., "Vitaminas y Sistema Nervioso," *Revista Clínica Española*, 1941b, Vol. 2, p. 209-232.

Grey, E., *The Food of Japan*, League of Nations, Geneva, 1928.

Handbook for the preparation of food balance sheets, FAO, Washington, 1949.

Health Organisation Report, League of Nations, Geneva, 1936, p. 6.

Hindende, M., "The Effect of Food Restriction During War on Mortality in Copenhagen," *Journal of the American Medical Association*, 1920, Vol. 74, No. 6.

"International standards for vitamin E," *League of Nations Bulletin of the Health organisation*, 1940/41, Vol. 9, p. 436-442.

Jiménez, F., Jiménez, M., "La alimentación en la provincia de Jaén. Deducciones sanitarias," in *Contribución al I Congreso Nacional de Sanidad del laboratorio de Higiene de la Alimentación y de la Nutrición y Técnica Bromatológica*, Escuela Nacional de Sanidad, Madrid, 1934, p. 25-34.

Jiménez, F., "Necesidades energéticas y dietéticas en la zona de Navalmoral de la Mata (Cáceres)," *Revista de Sanidad e Higiene Pública*, 1935, p. 470-477.

Jiménez García, F., "Estudio clínico de los trastornos carenciales observados en la población civil de Madrid durante la Guerra (1936-1939)," *Revista Clínica Española*, 1940, Vol. 1, p. 231-237.

Jiménez García, F., Grande Covián, F., "Sobre los trastornos carenciales observados en Madrid durante la Guerra. I. Los cuadros clínicos presentados con más frecuencia y su clasificación," *Revista Clínica Española*, 1940a, Vol. 1, p. 313-318.

Jiménez García, F., Grande Covián, F., "Algunas observaciones sobre las dietas consumidas por los enfermos carenciales de Madrid," *Revista Clínica Española*, 1940b, Vol. 1, No. 1.

Jiménez García, F., Grande Covián, F., "Sobre los trastornos carenciales observados en Madrid durante la Guerra. III. La presentación de los cuadros carenciales, en relación con la edad y el sexo de los pacientes," *Revista Clínica Española*, 1940, Vol. 1, p. 323-328.

Jiménez, F., Torres, T., "Las necesidades calóricas alimenticias de los internados en nuestras instituciones benéficas," in *Primer Congreso Nacional de Sanidad. Madrid, 6-12 de mayo de 1934*. Madrid, 1935, Vol. 4, p. 137-142.

Jiménez Díaz, C., *Estudios de nutrición*, Instituto de Investigaciones Médicas, Madrid, 1941-1943.

Kriegsernährungsplan für den Zeitraum 1.10.1938-1.8.1939. Teil I 1938, in BBAW, Institut für Ernährung, Historische Abteilung, No. 72.

Kusama, Y., Ochi, T., Higuchi, T., *Studies on the basal metabolism*. League of Nations, Geneva, 1937, 6 p. [C.H. 1256].

Lacaisse R., *L'Organisation d'Hygiène de la Société des Nations*, Société des Nations, Geneva, 1923.

Lacaisse R., *L'Hygiène internationale et la Société des Nations*, Éditions du 'Mouvement Sanitaire', Paris, 1926.

Laugier, H., "General Programme of Research into Biological Measurements and Tests for the Definition of States of Malnutrition," *League of Nations Quarterly Bulletin of the Health Organisation*, 1936, Vol. 5, No. 3, p. 505-530.

Lesné, E., Dreyfus-Sée, G., "Nutrition in childhood," *League of Nations Quarterly Bulletin of the Health Organisation*, 1936, Vol. 5, No. 3, p. 531-43.

Mackenzie, M.D., "The Administrative Machinery by which the Adequate Nourishment of the Poor is Ensured in Great Britain," *League of Nations Quarterly Bulletin of the Health Organisation*, 1933, Vol. 2, p. 333-352.

MacRae, T.F., "The adoption of crystalline vitamin B1 Hydrochloride as the new international standards of vitamin B1 and comparison of its potency with that of the former standard. A summary of Co-operative Experiments organised by the Accessory Food Factors Committee (Lister Institute and Medical Research Council)," *League of Nations Bulletin of the Health organisation*, 1940-1941, Vol. 9, p. 371-424.

Maestre Ibañez, M., *Doce conferencias de análisis de alimentos: guía práctica de análisis.* Sucesores de Rivadeneyra, Madrid, 1926.

Martínez García, F., "Trastornos nutritivos como causa de la mortalidad infantil. Peligros del calor," in *Conferencias radiadas por el médico jefe del Servicio Provincial de Puericultura durante el año 1938*, Instituto Provincial de Higiene de la Coruña "Al Servicio de España y del niño español," La Coruña, 1939, p. 5-9.

Martínez Vargas, A., "Selección de los niños 'pretuberculosos'. Ponencia al Congreso Nacional de Tuberculosis (Zaragoza, 1908)," *La Salud Pública. Revista de Higiene y Tuberculosis*, 1909, Vol. 5, p. 6-9.

[McDougall, E.J.] "Rural dietaries in Europe," *Bulletin of the Health Organisation*, 1939, Vol. 8, No. 3, p. 470-497. [C.H./Com.Exp.Alim./59, 25 p.].

"Memorandum prepared by the Health Section of the League of Nations: the Economic Depression and Public Health," *League of Nations Quarterly Bulletin of the Health Organisation*, 1932, Vol. 1, p. 425.

"Memorandum on the International Standard for vitamin E from the Department of Biological Standards, nationa Institute of medical Research. (Lister Institute and Medical Research Council)," *League of Nations Quarterly Bulletin of the Health Organisation*, 1940-1941, Vol. 9, p. 443-446.

Methodology of diet surveys, FAO, Washington, 1948.

"Milk Problem, The," *League of Nations Bulletin of the Health Organisation*, 1937, Vol. 6, No. 2, p. 371-504.

Milk Problem. A Critical Study of its Nutritional, Hygienic, Economic and Social Aspects by HC Bendixen, GJ Blink, JC Drummond, AM Leroy, GS Wilson, League of Nations, Geneva, 1937.

Moerkeberg, H.C., *Meat inspection in Denmark and Inspection of Milk in Denmark*, League of Nations, Geneva, 1924. [C.H./E.P.S./49].

Moreno Luque, J., *Algunas normas sobre alimentación humana y sobre Economía, Agrícola, Ganadera y Forestal estudiadas durante su cautiverio en Madrid*, Prólogo de José Mª Fernández-Ladreda, Madrid, 1939.

Moroder, J., "Los puntos de vista sanitarios de la alimentación humana," *Revista de Sanidad e Higiene Pública*, 1934, p. 167-175.

"Most Suitable Methods of Detecting Malnutrition Due to the Economic Depression, The. Conference held at Berlin from December 5th to 7th, 1932," *League of Nations Quarterly Bulletin of the Health Organisation*, 1933, Vol. 1, p. 116-129.

Muehel, W., "Ill effects of food restrictions in Europe, 1940-1944," *League of Nations Bulletin of the Health Organisation*, 1945-1946, Vol. 12.

Nobécourt, P., Vitry, G., "Clinical methods for determining the state of nutrition in school children," *League of Nations Quarterly Bulletin of the Health Organisation*, 1936, Vol. 5, No. 3, p. 544-48.

Noguer-Moré, J., *Nuestra alimentación en tiempos de escasez*, Biblioteca Hygia, Barcelona, 1937.

Nutrition: the newer diagnostic methods. Proceedings of the round table on nutrition and public health, Milbank Memorial Fund, New York, 1938.

Nutrition in various countries, Series of League of Nations Publications, Geneva, 1936. [Technical Report A.12(b).1936.II.B].

Olmeda Viorreta, C., "Contribución al estudio vitamínico de los alimentos españoles. Experiencias llevadas a cabo entre 1934 y 1935," *Revista de Sanidad e Higiene Pública*, 1936, Vol. 11, No. 3, p. 205-231.

Orr J.B., *The influence of nutrition on the incidence of disease*, Hudson and Son, London, 1925.

Orr J.B., *Food, Health & Income: Report on a Survey of Adequacy of Diet in Relation to Income*, Macmillan & Co, London, 1936.

Orr J.B., *The role of food in post-war reconstruction*, International Labour Organisation, Geneva, 1943.

Palanca y Martínez Fortún, J. A., "Rapport sur la situation épidémiologique de l'Espagne pendant l'année 1939," Société des Nations, Genève, 1939, p. 40-52.

Palanca y Martínez Fortún, J. A., *Les services sanitaires espagnols pendant la guerre civile*, Société de Nations, Genève, 1939.

Peraita, M., "Sobre el tratamiento por el ácido nicotínico de los síntomas nerviosos y mentales de los pelagrosos," *Revista de Sanidad e Higiene Pública*, 1940, p. 482-503.

Pi i Sunyer, A., *El hambre de los pueblos.* Conferencia dada por el Doctor. Augusto Pi i Sunyer en la Academia de Medicina en 29 de enero de 1922, Asociación instructiva de obreros y empleados municipales, Barcelona, 1922.

Pi i Sunyer Bayo, J., *Principis generals de dietética*, Monografies Mèdiques, Barcelona, 1930.

Pittaluga, G., *El problema de las vitaminas y la alimentación del obrero*, Sociedad Española de Higiene, Madrid, 1917.

Pittaluga, G., *La constitución de la Escuela Nacional de Sanidad de Madrid (España)*, Escuela Nacional de Sanidad, Madrid, 1930.

Problem of nutrition. Interim Report of the Mixed Committee on the Problem of Nutrition, 3 vols, League of Nations, Geneva, 1936. [A.12.1936.II.B].

Pulido, A., "Prólogo," in Ubeda y Correal, J., *El presupuesto de la familia obrera*, Dirección General de Sanidad (Monografías), Madrid, 1902, p. 7-8.

Puche Alvarez, J., "El hambre en Europa," *Ciencia (México)*, 1940, Vol. 1, 6 p.

Randoin, L., "On the necessity for a biological supervision of food (with Special Reference to its Vitamin Content)," *League of Nations Quarterly Bulletin of the Health Organisation*, 1936, Vol. 5, No. 3, p. 493-504.

Rapport sur la mission sanitaire en Espagne (28 décembre 1936-15 janvier 1937), Société des Nations, Genève, 1937, 62 p.

Rationnement alimentaire et ravitaillement 1943-1944, Société des Nations, Genève, 1944.

Raventós, J., *L'Alimentació humana*, Mancomunitat de Catalunya (Publicacions divulgadores dels Serveis Tècnics d'Agricultura, núm. 8), Barcelona, 1923.

Relation of Nutrition to Health, Agriculture and Economy Policy, The Final Report of the Mixed Committee of the League of Nations, League of Nations, Geneva, 1937.

Report on the food requirements of man, Food war committee, Royal Society, London, 1919.

"Report on the Best Methods of Safeguarding the Public Health during the Depression," *League of Nations Quarterly Bulletin of the Health Organisation*, 1933, Vol. 2, p. 286-332.

"Report on the Physiological Bases of Nutrition by the Technical Commission of the Health Committee in the meeting held in London November 25th-29th, 1935," *League of Nations Quarterly Bulletin of the Health Organisation*, 1936, Vol. 5, No. 3, p. 391-415.

"Report of the Health Organisation for the Period October 1932 to September 1933. IV. Economic Depression and Public Health," *League of Nations Quarterly Bulletin of the Health Organisation*, 1933, Vol. 2, p. 529-535.

"Report by the Technical Commission on Nutrition on the work of its second session held in Geneva, June 4th to 8th, 1936," *League of Nations Quarterly Bulletin of the Health Organisation*, 1936, Vol. 5, No. 3, p. 416-426.

"Report on the work of the group of experts appointed to study methods of assession the state of nutrition in infants and adolescents," *League of Nations Bulletin of the Health Organisation*, 1937, Vol. 6, No. 2, p. 129-204.

"Report by the Technical Commission on Nutrition on the Work of its third session, held in London from November 15th to 20th, 1937," *Bulletin of the Health Organisation*, 1938, Vol. 7, p. 460-502.

"Report on the Meeting of Directors of Institutes and Schools of Hygiene held in Geneva from November 22nd to 27th, 1937. F. Nutrition," *League of Nations Bulletin of the Health Organisation*, 1938, Vol. 7, p. 186-190.

"Report on the work of the Health Organisation between June 1937 and May 1938, and on its 1938 Programme. 4. Nutrition," *League of Nations Bulletin of the Health Organisation*, 1938, Vol. 7, p. 642-647.

"Report on the work of the Health Organisation between June 1938 and April 1939 and on its 1939 programme. B. Nutrition," *League of Nations Bulletin of the Health Organisation*, 1939, Vol. 8, p. 27-32.

"Report on Bread in several European Countries," *League of Nations Bulletin of the Health organisation*, 1939, Vol. 8, p. 498-550.

Richet, Ch., "The nutritional requirements of puberty," *League of Nations Quarterly Bulletin of the Health Organisation*, 1936, Vol. 5, No. 3, p. 549-553.

Richet, Ch., *Alimentación y regímenes alimentarios*, Espasa-Calpe, Madrid, 1942.

Robinson, W. D., Janney, J. H., Grande (Covián), F., "An Evaluation of the Nutritional Status of a Population Group in Madrid, Spain, during the Summer of 1941," *Journal of Nutrition*, 1942, Vol. 24, No. 6, p. 557-584.

Rockefeller Foundation, *Report on the health situation in Spain*, Rockefeller Archive Centre, New York, 20 August 1939.

Rodríguez Abaytúa, R., *Bioenergética y termoquímica alimenticia: estudio razonado para la alimentación del adulto*, Nicolás Moya, Madrid, 1921.

Rof Carballo, J., Grande Covián, F., "Calambres musculares como síntomas carenciales," *Revista Clínica Española*, 1943, Vol. 8.

Rosell, J. M., *Los actuales conocimientos del metabolismo mineral: la importancia fisiológica, patológica, terapéutica e higiénica de los elementos minerales contenidos en los alimentos y en el agua*, Barcelona, 1927.

Ruiz Gijón, J., *El diagnóstico de la pelagra por el laboratorio*, J. Cosano, Madrid, 1941.

Ruiz Gijón, J., *Estudio de las relaciones entre el metabolismo de la creatina y el de los hidratos de carbono*, J. Cosano, Madrid, 1942.

"Rural Dietaries in Europe," *League of Nations Bulletin of the Health organisation*, 1939, Vol. 8, p. 470-497.

Saiki T., *Progress of the Science of Nutrition in Japan*, League of Nations, Geneva, 1926.

Saiki T., *Necessity of the Study of Nutrition*, League of Nations, Geneva, 1927.

Sanidad Nacional. Disposiciones oficiales emanadas del Ministerio de la Gobernación (Dirección General de Sanidad), 32 vols, Ministerio de la Gobernación, Madrid, 1903-1935.

Schiötz, C., *Appreciation de l'etat de nutrition des enfants. Remarques préliminaires*, League of Nations, Geneva, 1936.

"Second Conference on Vitamin Standardisation," *League of Nations Quarterly Bulletin of the Health Organisation*, 1934, Vol. 3, p. 428-440.

"Second General Report on certain European Schools and Institutes of Hygiene. 5. School of Health and National Institute of Hygiene, Madrid," *League of Nations Bulletin of the Health Organisation*, (1938), Vol. VII, p. 309-312.

"Standardisation of certain methods used in making dietary studies. Conference of experts held in Rome," *League of Nations Quarterly Bulletin of the Health Organisation*, 1932, Vol. 1, p. 477.

Tarralluela i Albareda, J., *Higiene de l'alimentació*, Minerva, Diputación de Barcelona, Barcelona, 1919.

"Technical Commission on Nutrition. Report by a Special Committee which met in Geneva from August 22nd to 24th, 1938," *Bulletin of the Health Organisation*, 1938, Vol. 7, p. 667-678.

Terroine, E.F., "The Protein Component in the Human Diet," *League of Nations Quarterly Bulletin of the Health Organisation*, 1936, Vol. 5, No. 3, p. 427-492.

Úbeda y Correal, J., *El presupuesto de la familia obrera*, Dirección General de Sanidad, Madrid, 1902.

Veen, A.G. van, "The rice problem," *League of Nations Bulletin of the Health Organisation*, 1940, Vol. 9, p. 357-60.

Voit, C. von, *Food and the Principles of Dietetics*, London, 1927.

Worker's nutrition and social policy, League of Nations, Geneva, 1936.

Selected bibliography

Amrith S., "Development and Disease: Public Health and the United Nations, c. 1945-55," in Daunton M., Trentmann F. (eds.), *Worlds of Political Economy. Knowledge and Power in the Nineteenth and Twentieth Centuries*, Palgrave Macmillan, Basingstoke, p. 221-250.

Andresen, A., Elvbakken. K.T., Hubbard, W. (eds.), *Public Health and Preventive Medicine 1800-2000*, Stein Rokkan Centre for Social Studies, Bergen, Report 1-2004.

Andresen A., Grønlie T., Ryymin T. (eds.), *Science, Culture and Politics. European Perspectives on Medicine, Sickness and Health*, Stein Rokkan Centre for Social Studies, Bergen, 2006.

Andresen A., Grønlie T., Ryymin T. (eds.), *Transferring Medico-Political Knowledge in Nineteenth- and Twentieth-Century Europe*, Rokkan Centre for Social Studies, Bergen, 2007.

Andresen, A., Barona, J.L., Cherry, S. (eds.), *Making a new countryside? Health Policies and Practices in European History c. 1860-1950*, Peter Lang, Frankfurt, 2009.

Apple R. D., *Vitamania: Vitamins in American Culture*, New Brunswick, New York, 1996.

Apple, R. D., "Vitamins win the war: nutrition, commerce, and patriotism in the United States during the Second World War," in Smith, D.F., Phillips, J. (eds.), *Food, Science, Policy and Regulation in the Twentieth Century: International and Comparative Perspectives*, Routledge, London, 2000, p. 135-150.

Badger Anthony, J., *The New Deal. The Depression Years 1933-1940*, Hill and Wang, New York, 1989.

Baldwin, P., *The Politics of Social Solidarity. Class Bases of the European Welfare State 1875-1975*, Cambridge University Press, Cambridge, 1990.

Barnes, G. N., *History of the International Labour Office*, Williams and Norgate, London, 1926.

Barnes, D.S., *The Great Stink of Paris and the Nineteenth-Century Struggle against Filth and Germs*, The Johns Hopkins University Press, Baltimore, 2006.

Barona J. L., "Rural Life and the Problem of Nutrition. Technical Approaches by the Nutrition Committee of the League of Nations," in Andresen A., Grønlie T., Ryymin T. (eds.), *Science, Culture and Politics. European Perspectives on Medicine, Sickness and Health*, Stein Rokkan Centre for Social Studies, Bergen, 2006, p. 201-14.

Barona, J. L., "Nutrition, knowledge, and action. International trends and social policies in Spain, 1931-1944," in Andersen, A., Gronlie, T. (eds.), *Transferring Medico-Political Knowledge in 19th and 20th Century Europe*, Stein Rokkan Centre for Social Studies, Bergen, 2007a, p. 91-108.

Barona, J. L., “La salud de la población según los informes internacionales,” in *Actas del Congreso Internacional sobre la Guerra Civil Española*, Sociedad Estatal de Conmemoraciones Culturales, Madrid, 2007b.

Barona J. L., “Nutrition and Health. The International Context during the Interwar Crisis,’ *Social History of Medicine*, 2008a, Vol. 21, No. 1, p. 87-105.

Barona, J. L., “International Organisations and the Development of a Physiology of Nutrition during the 1930s,” *Food and History*, 2008b, Vol. 6, No. 1.

Barona, J. L., Cherry S., *Health and Medicine in Rural Europe (1850-1945)*, Seminari d’Estudis sobre la Ciència, Universitat de València, València, 2005.

Barona, J. L., Bernabeu-Mestre, J., Perdiguero, E., “Health Problems and Public Policies in Rural Spain (1854-1936),” in Barona, J. L., Cherry S., *Health and Medicine in Rural Europe (1850-1945)*, Seminari d’Estudis sobre la Ciència, Universitat de València, València, 2005, p. 63-82.

Barona, J. L., Perdiguero E., “Health and the War. Changing schemes and health conditions during the Spanish Civil War,” *Dynamis*, 2008, Vol. 28, p. 103-123.

Beneito, A., Puche Gil, J., “Creixement econòmic i desenvolupament fabril en Alcoi, 1840-1915: Misèria fisiològica sota l’esplendor industrial?,” in *La societat industrial al País Valencià*, Alcoi, 2008.

Bengoa Lecanda, J.M., *Tras la ruta del hambre. Nutrición y salud pública en el siglo XX*, Publicaciones Universidad de Alicante, Alicante, 2007.

Bengoa Lecanda, JM., “Historia de la nutrición en salud pública,” in Serra Majem, L. *et al.*, *Nutrición y salud pública. Métodos, bases científicas y aplicaciones*, Masson, Barcelona, 2006, p. 52-61.

Bennett, J., *The Hunger Machine: The Politics of Food*, Politi, Cambridge, 1987.

Berkov, R., *The World Health organisation: A Study in Decentralised Internacional Administration*, Librarie E. Droz, Geneva, 1957.

Bernabeu-Mestre, J. *et al.*, “La alimentación como problema sanitario: nutrición y salud pública en la España de la primera mitad del siglo XX,” in *VIII Congreso de la ADEH*, Maó, 2007, 63 p.

Bernabeu-Mestre, J. *et al.*, *Investigación e innovación tecnológica en la ciencia de la nutrición. El abordaje de la malnutrición en el contexto de la cultura científica*, Editorial Club Universitario, Alicante, 2008.

Bernabeu-Mestre, J. *et al.*, “Nutrition and public health in the contemporary Spain, 1900-1936,” *Food and History*, 2008, Vol. 6, No. 1.

Bernabeu-Mestre, J., Galiana, M.E., Esplugues, J.X. and Cid, P., “Overexploitation, malnutrition and stigma in a women’s illness: chlorosis in contemporary Spanish medicine (1877-1936),” in Harris, B., Gálvez, L., Machado, E. (eds.), *Gender and wellbeing in Europe: historical and contemporary perspectives*, Ashgate, Hampshire, 2009, p. 154-171.

Blecourt, W., Usbourne, C. (eds.), *Cultural Approaches to the History of Medicine. Mediating Medicine in Early Modern and Modern Europe*, Palgrave, Basingstoke, 2004.

Bonzon, T., "Consumption and total Warfare in Paris (1914-1918)," in Trentman F., Just F. (eds.), *Food and Conflict in Europe in the Age of the Two World Wars*, Palgrave, New York, 2006, p. 49-64.

Borowy, I., Grüner, W.D. (eds.), *Facing Illness in Troubled Times. Health in Europe in the Interwar Years 1918-1939*, Peter Lang, Frankfurt am Main, 2005.

Brassley, P., Potter, A., "A view From the Top: Social Elites and Food Consumption in Britain, 1930s-1940s," in Trentman F. and Just F. (eds.), *Food and Conflict in Europe in the Age of the Two World Wars*, Palgrave, New York, 2006, p. 223-242.

Brunton, D. (ed.), *Medicine Transformed: Health, Disease and Society in Europe 1800-1930*, Manchester University/Open University Press, Manchester, 2004.

Calandre, C., "El Dr. Luis Calandre Ibáñez. Su actuación en la Guerra Civil Española (1937-1939)," *Frente de Madrid*, 2007, Vol. 11, p. 6-11.

Cannon, G., *The Politics of Food*, London, 1988.

Caplan, P. (ed.), *Food, Health and Identity*, Routledge, London, 1997.

Contreras Hernández, J., Gracia Arnáiz, M., *Alimentación y cultura. Perspectivas antropológicas*, Ariel, Barcelona, 2005.

Corni, G., Horst G., *Brot – Butter- Kanonen. Die Ernährungswirtschaft in Deutschland unter der Diktatur Hitlers*, Berlin, 1994.

Crawford E., *Nationalism and Internationalism in Science, 1880-1939*, Cambridge University Press, Cambridge, 1992.

Cullather, N., "The Foreign Policy of the Calorie," *The American Historical Review*, 2007, Vol. 112, p. 337-364.

Cura, M.I. del, Huertas, R., *Alimentación y enfermedad en tiempos de hambre. España, 1937-1947*, Consejo Superior de Investigaciones Cientificas, Madrid, 2007.

Cussó Segura, X., "Estado nutritivo de la población española, 1900-1970: análisis de las necesidades y disponibilidades de nutrientes," *Revista de Agricultura e Historia Rural*, 2005, Vol. 36, p. 329-358.

Cussò Segura, X., Garrobou, R., "La transición nutricional en la España contemporánea: las variaciones en el consumo de pan, patatas y legumbres," *Investigaciones de Historia Económica*, 2007, Vol. 7, p. 69-100.

Daunton M., Hilton M. (eds.), *The Politics of Consumption: Material Culture and Citizenship in Europe and America*, Oxford, 2001.

Daunton M., Trentmann F. (eds.), *Worlds of Political Economy. Knowledge and Power in the Nineteenth and Twentieth Centuries*, Palgrave Macmillan, Basingstoke, 2006.

Davis B. J., *Home Fires Burning: Food, Politics and Everyday Life in World War I Berlin*, NC, Chapel Hill, 2000.

Davis R., Wheatcroft S., *The Years of Hunger*, Palgrave, Basingstoke, 2004.

Dinter, A., *Berlin in Trümmern. Ernährungslage und medizinische Versorgung der Bevölkerung Berlins nach dem II. Weltkrieg*, Berlin, 1999.

Dubin, M., "The League of Nations Health Organization," in Weindling, P. (ed.), *International health organisations and movements, 1918-1939*, Cambridge University Press, Cambridge, 1995. p. 56-80.

Elvbakken, K. T., Lægreid, P., Rykkja, L. H., "Regulation for Safe Food; a Comparison of Five European Countries," *Scandinavian Political Studies*, 2008, Vol. 31, No. 2, p. 125-148.

Freeman, R., *The Politics of Health in Europe*, Manchester University Press, Manchester, 2000.

French, M., Phillips J., "Compositional food standards in the United Kingdom: the case of the Willis Inquiry, 1929-1934," in Smith, D. F., Phillips J., *Food, Science, Policy and Regulation in the Twentieth Century. International and Comparative Perspectives*, Routledge, London, 2000, p. 17-36.

Galius M., Volkmann H., *Der Kampf um das tägliche Brot: Nahrungsmangel, Versorgungspolitik und Protest, 1770-1990*, Opladen, 1994.

García-Albea Ristol E., "Las neuropatías carenciales en Madrid durante la Guerra Civil," *Neurología*, 1999, Vol. 14, p. 122-129.

Gracia Arnaiz, M., *Somos lo que comemos. Estudios de alimentación y cultura en España*, Ariel Antropología, Barcelona, 2002.

Gracia Arnaiz M., Comelles J.M. (eds.), *No comerás. Narrativas sobre comida, cuerpo y género en el nuevo milenio*, Icaria, Observatorio de la Alimentación, Barcelona, 2007.

Gratzer, W., *Terrors of the Table: The Curious History of Nutrition*, Oxford University Press, Oxford, 2005.

Gries, R., *Die Rationen-Gesellschaft. Versorgungskampf und Vergleichsmentalität: Leipzig, München und Köln nach dem Kriege*, Münster, 1991.

Guillem-Llobat, X., Perdiguero, E., "Fighting adulteration in early European food industrialisation. The case of Alicante (Spain)," in Vámos, É. (ed.), *History of the Food Chain. From Agriculture to Consumption and Waste*, Hungarian Chemical Society, Budapest, 2006a, p. 33-40.

Guillem-Llobat, X., "Industrialització i alimentació en la societat valenciana. El control de qualitat dels aliments (1850-1939)," in Herran, N. *et al.* (eds.), *Synergia: Primer Encuentro de Jóvenes Investigadores en Historia de la Ciencia*, Consejo Superior de Investigaciones Cientificas, Madrid, 2006b.

Guillem-Llobat, X., *El control de la qualitat dels aliments. El cas valencià en el context internacional (1878-1936)*, PUV, Valencia, 2007.

Guillem-Llobat, X., "El control dels aliments. Una perspectiva històrica," *L'Espill*, 2008a, Vol. 29, p. 153-157.

Guillem-Llobat, X., "El establecimiento de nuevos límites de calidad para los alimentos en el cambio de siglo (1880-1936)," in Ortiz Gomez, T. *et al.* (eds.), *La Experiencia de enfermar en perspectiva histórica. Actas XIV Con-*

greso de la Sociedad Española de Historia de la Medicina, Editorial Universidad de Granada, Granada, 2008b, p. 271-274.

Guillem-Llobat, X., "El paper dels laboratoris municipals valencians en el control de qualitat dels aliments (1881-1936)," *Actes del Congrès de la Societat Catalana d'Història de la Ciència i de la Tècnica*, 2008c, Vol. 1, p. 293-300.

Guillem-Llobat, X., "Food quality controls in the European Periphery. Valencian scientists and laboratories in the late nineteenth century," in Simon, J. *et al.* (eds.), *Beyond Borders: Fresh perspectives in history of science*, Cambridge Scholars Publishing, Cambridge, 2008d, p. 301-324.

Harrison, M., *Disease and the Modern World*, Polity, Cambridge, 2004.

Heim, S., *Kalorien, Kautschuk, Karrieren. Pflanzenzüchtung und landwirtschaftliche Forschung in Kaiser-Wilhelm-Instituten 1933-1945*, Göttingen, 2003.

Hendrick, H., *Child Welfare. Historical Dimension, Contemporary Debate*, Polity Press, Cambridge, 2003.

Hobsbawn, E., *The Age of Extremes, 1914-1991*, Abacus, London, 1995.

Horrocks, S.M., "Nutrition Science and the Food and Pharmaceutical Industries in Inter-war Britain," in Smith, D.F. (ed.), *Nutrition in Britain. Science, Scientisits and Politics in the Twentieth Century*, Routledge, London & Nueva York, 1997, p. 53-74.

Kamminga H., Cunningham A., *The Science and Culture of Nutrition (1840-1940)*, Rodopi, Amsterdam, 1997.

Kamminga H., "Axes to grind": popularising the science of vitamins, 1920s and 1930s," in Smith D. F., Phillips J., *Food, Science, Policy and Regulation in the Twentieth Century. International and Comparative Perspectives*, Routledge, London, 2000, p. 83-100.

Langreo, A., Pujol Andreu, J., "Evolución económica agroalimentaria," in *Como vivíamos: alimentos y alimentación en la España del siglo XX*, Lunwerg, Madrid, 2007, p. 41-66.

Livi-Bacci, M., *Population and Nutrition: An Essay on European Demographic History*, Cambridge University Press, Cambridge, 1991.

López Núñez, A., *Los inicios de la protección a la infancia en España*, Madrid, 1992.

Löwy, I., Krigge, J. (eds.), *Images of Disease. Science, Public Policy and Health in Post-war Europe*, Office for Official Publications of the European Communities, Luxembourg, 2001.

Ludvigsen, K., Elvbakken K. T., *The Public, the Mother and the Child. Public Health Initiatives Promoting the Strong and Happy Child - Focusing on Food and Mental Health*, Rokkan Centre for Social Studies, Bergen, 2005.

Marchisio, S., Di Blasé A., *The Food and Agriculture Organization*, Dordrecht, 1991.

Maier, C. S., "Between Taylorism and Technocracy: European Ideologies and the Vision of Industrial Productivity in the 1920s," *Journal of Contemporary History*, 1970, Vol. 5, p. 27-61.

Martínez Carrión, J.M., "Biología, historia y medio ambiente: la estatura como espejo del nivel de vida de la sociedad española," *Ayer*, 2002, Vol. 46, p. 93-122.

Martínez Carrión, J.M., "El nivel de vida en la España rural. Siglos XVIII-XX. Nuevos enfoques, nuevos resultados," in Martínez Carrión, J.M., Pérez Castejón, J.J. (eds.), *El nivel de vida en la España rural, siglos XVIII-XX*, Universidad de Alicante, Alicante, p. 15-72.

Maurer, D., Sobal J. (eds.), *Eating Agendas: Food and Nutrition as Social Problems*, New York, 1995.

Milward, A., Saul, S. B., *The Development of the Economies of Continental Europe*, Allen and Unwin, London, 1977.

Nicolau Nos, R., Pujol Andreu, J., "El consumo de proteínas animales en Barcelona entre las décadas de 1830 y 1930: evolución y factores condicionantes," *Investigaciones de Historia Económica*, 2005a, Vol. 3, p. 101-134.

Nicolau Nos, R., Pujol Andreu, J., "Variaciones regionales de los precios de consumo y de las dietas en España, en los inicios de la transición demográfica," *Documents de Treball (UAB. Unitat d'Història Econòmica)*, 2005b, No. 29.

Nicolau Nos, R., Pujol Andreu, J., "Alimentación, beneficencia y condiciones de vida en la transformación de las zonas rurales durante la industrialización: Olot, siglos XIX-XX," *Documents de Treball (UAB. Unitat d'Història Econòmica)*, 2005b, No. 30.

Nicolau Nos, R., Pujol Andreu, J., "Los factores condicionantes de la transición nutricional en la Europa Occidental: Barcelona, 1890-1936," *Scripta Nova: Revista Electrónica de Geografía y Ciencias Sociales*, 2008, Vol. 12, p. 256-265.

Nijs, T. de, "Food Retailing in The Hague, 1914-1930," in Trentman F. and Just F. (eds.), *Food and Conflict in Europe in the Age of the Two World Wars*, Palgrave, New York, 2006, p. 65-87.

Nützenadel, A., "Dictating Food: Autarchy, Food Provision, and Consumer Politics in Fascist Italy, 1922-1943," in Trentman F. and Just F. (eds.), *Food and Conflict in Europe in the Age of the Two World Wars*, Palgrave, New York, 2006, p. 88-108.

Perdiguero, E., "On Food. The popularization of nutrition in Internar Spain," in Andresen, A., Gronlie, T. (eds.), *Transferring Medico-Political Knowledge in 19th and 20th-Century Europe*, Bergen, Stein Rokkan Centre for Social Studies, 2007.

Perdiguero, E. (ed.), *Salvad al niño. La protección a la infancia en los países de la Europa mediterránea*, Seminari d'Estudis sobre la Ciencia, Universitat de València, Valencia, 2005.

Phillips, R. W., *FAO, its Origins, Formation and Evolution 1945-1981*, FAO, Rome, 1981.

Porter, D. (ed.), *The History of Public Health and the Modern State*, Rodopi, Amsterdam, 1994.

Porter, R. (ed.), *The Popularisation of Medicine 1650-1850*, Routledge, London, 1992.

Roodhouse, M., "Popular Morality and the Black Market in Britain, 1939-1955," in Trentman F. and Just F. (eds.), *Food and Conflict in Europe in the Age of the Two World Wars*, Palgrave, New York, 2006, p. 243-265.

Rosen, G., *A History of Public Health. Introduction by Elizabeth Fee: Biographical Essay and New Bibliography by Edward T. Morman*, Johns Hopkins University Press, Baltimore, 1993.

Rosenberg, E. S., *Financial Missionaries to the World: The Politics and Culture of Dollar Diplomacy, 1900-1930*, Harvard University Press, Cambridge MA, 1999.

Rotberg, R.I., Raab, T.K., *Hunger and History. The Impact of Changing Food Production and Consumption Patterns of Society*, Cambridge University Press, Cambridge, 1985.

Ruxin, J., "The United Nations Protein Advisory Group," in Smith, D.F., Phillips, J. (eds.), *Food, Science, Policy and Regulation in the Twentieth Century: International and Comparative Perspectives*, Routledge, London, 2000, p. 151-166.

Ryymin, T., "Tuberculosis-threatened Children. The Rise and Fall of a Medical Concept, *c.* 1900-60," in Andresen A., Grønlie T., Ryymin T. (eds.), *Transferring Medico-Political Knowledge in Nineteenth- and Twentieth-Century Europe*, Rokkan Centre for Social Studies, Bergen, 2007.

Ryymin T., "Tuberculosis-threatened Children. The Rise and Fall of a Medical Concept in Norway, *c.* 1900-60," *Medical History*, 2008, Vol. 52, p. 347-364.

Sabaté y Cañellas, F., "Las encuestas de alimentación y nutrición en España. Bibliografía 1939-1979," *Revista de Sanidad e Higiene Pública*, 1984, Vol. 58, p. 117-1132.

Scott J. C., *Seeing like a State: How Certain Schemes to Improve the Human Condition Have Failed*, Yale University Press, New Haven, 1998.

Sen, A.K., *Poverty and Famines. An Essay on Entitlement and Deprivation*, Oxford University Press, Oxford, 1981.

Simón Pérez, H., J. Escudero, A., "El bienestar en España: una perspectiva de largo plazo, 1850-1991," *Revista de Historia Económica*, 2003, Vol. 2, p. 525-566.

Slater, D., *Consumer Culture and Modernity*, Cambridge, 1997.

Smith, D.F. (ed.), *Nutrition in Britain: Science, Scientists and Politics in the Twentieth Century*, London and New York, 1997.

Smith, D. F., Phillips J. (eds.), *Food, Science, Policy and Regulation in the Twentieth Century. International and Comparative Perspectives*, Routledge, London, 2000.

Smith, D.F., "The rise and fall of the Scientific Food Committee during the Second World War," in Smith, D. F., Phillips J. (eds.), *Food, Science, Policy and Regulation in the Twentieth Century. International and Comparative Perspectives*, Routledge, London, 2000, p. 101-116.

Spiekermann, U., "Brown Bread for Victory: German and British Wholemeal Politics in the Inter-War Period," in Trentman F. and Just F. (eds.), *Food and Conflict in Europe in the Age of the Two World Wars*, Palgrave, New York, 2006, p. 143-171.

Staples, A. L. S., *The Birth of Development. How the World Bank, Food and Agriculture Organization, and World Health Organisation Changed the World, 1945-1965*, The Kent State University Press, Kent, 2006.

Steckel, R. H., Rose J. C. (eds.), *The Backbone of History. Health and Nutrition in the Western Hemisphere*, Cambridge University Press, Cambridge, 2002.

Tauger, M., "Stalin, Soviet Agriculture, and Collectivisation," in Trentman F. and Just F. (eds.), *Food and Conflict in Europe in the Age of the Two World Wars*, Palgrave, New York, 2006, p. 109-142.

Thoms, U., "Learning from America? The travels of German nutritional scientist to the USA in the Context of the technical Assistance Program of the Mutual Security Agencies and its consequences for West German Nutritional Policy," *Food and History*, 2004, Vol. 2, p. 117-151.

Trentman F., Just F. (eds.), *Food and Conflict in Europe in the Age of the Two World Wars*, Palgrave, New York, 2006.

Trentmann, F., "Coping with Shortage: The Problem of Food Security and Global Visions of Coordination, *c.* 1890s-1950," in Trentman F., Just F. (eds.), *Food and Conflict in Europe in the Age of the Two World Wars*, Palgrave, New York, 2006, p. 13-48.

Trittel, G., *Hunger und Politik. Die Ernährungskrise in der Bizone (1945-1949)*, Frankfurt, New York, 1990.

Velasco, C., Rodergas, R., "Los productos alimenticios y la publicidad," in *Como vivíamos: alimentos y alimentación en la España del siglo XX*, Lunwerg, Madrid, 2007, p. 119-138.

Vernon J., "The Ethics of Hunger and the Assembly of Society: The Techno-Politics of the School Meal in Modern Britain," *American Historical Review*, 2005, Vol. 110, p. 693-725.

Viaje a las Hurdes. El manuscrito inédito de Gregorio Marañón y las fotografías de la visita de Alfonso XIII, Madrid, El País-Aguilar, 1993.

Weindling, P., "Social Medicine at the League of Nations Health Organisation and the International Labour Office Compared," in Weindling P. (ed.), *International Health Organisations and Movements, 1918-1939*, Cambridge University Press, Cambridge, 1995a, 134-53.

Weindling, P., "The Role of International Organizations in Setting Nutritional Standards in the 1920s and 1930s," *Clio Médica*, 1995b, Vol. 32, p. 319-332.

Weindling, P., "Health and Medicine in Interwar Europe," in Cooter, R., Pickstone, J. (eds.), *Companion to Medicine in the Twentieth Century*, London, 2003, p. 29-50.

Weindling, P.J., *Nazi Medicine and the Nuremberg Trials: From Medical War Crimes to Informed Consent*, Palgrave Macmillan, New York, 2005.

Wolf, J. H., *Don't Kill your Baby: Public Health and the Decline of Breastfeeding in the Nineteenth and Twentieth Centuries*, Ohio University Press, Columbus, 2001.

Worboys, M., "The Discovery of Colonial Malnutrition between the Wars," in Arnold D. (ed.), *Imperial Medicine and Indigenous Society*, Manchester University Press, Manchester, 1988, p. 208-225.

Worboys, M., *Spreading Germs: Disease, Theories, and Medical Practice in Britain, 1865-1900*, Cambridge University Press, New York, 2000.